Frequently Asked Questions

# ORAL MEDICINE AND RADIOLOGY

## Frequently Asked Questions

# ORAL MEDICINE AND RADIOLOGY

*A free companion to Essential Quick Review: Oral Medicine and Radiology*

*Editor-in-Chief*

**Priya Verma Gupta** MDS FPFA
Professor
Department of Pedodontics and Preventive Dentistry
Divya Jyoti College of Dental Sciences and Research
Ghaziabad, Uttar Pradesh, India

*Co-Author*

**Jyoti Gupta** BDS MDS
Professor
Department of Oral Medicine and Radiology
Career Post Graduate Institution of Dental Science and Hospital
Lucknow, Uttar Pradesh, India

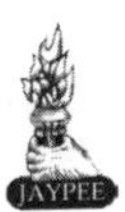

*The Health Sciences Publisher*

New Delhi | London | Philadelphia | Panama

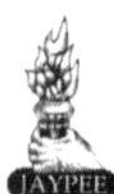

**Jaypee Brothers Medical Publishers (P) Ltd**

**Headquarters**
Jaypee Brothers Medical Publishers (P) Ltd
4838/24, Ansari Road, Daryaganj
New Delhi 110 002, India
Phone: +91-11-43574357
Fax: +91-11-43574314
Email: jaypee@jaypeebrothers.com

**Overseas Offices**

J.P. Medical Ltd
83 Victoria Street, London
SW1H 0HW (UK)
Phone: +44 20 3170 8910
Fax: +44 (0)20 3008 6180
Email: info@jpmedpub.com

Jaypee-Highlights Medical Publishers Inc.
City of Knowledge, Bld. 235, Clayton
Panama City, Panama
Phone: +1 507-301-0496
Fax: +1 507-301-0499
Email: cservice@jphmedical.com

Jaypee Medical Inc.
325 Chestnut Street
Suite 412, Philadelphia,
PA 19106, USA
Phone: +1 267-519-9789
Email: support@jpmedus.com

Jaypee Brothers Medical Publishers (P) Ltd
17/1-B Babar Road, Block-B, Shaymali
Mohammadpur, Dhaka-1207
Bangladesh
Mobile: +08801912003485
Email: jaypeedhaka@gmail.com

Jaypee Brothers Medical Publishers (P) Ltd
Bhotahity, Kathmandu, Nepal
Phone: +977-9741283608
Email: kathmandu@jaypeebrothers.com

Website: www.jaypeebrothers.com
Website: www.jaypeedigital.com



**Inquiries for bulk sales may be solicited at:** jaypee@jaypeebrothers.com

***Frequently Asked Questions: Oral Medicine and Radiology***

*First Edition*: **2016**

ISBN: 978-93-86107-79-4

*Printed at* Rajkamal Electric Press, Plot No. 2, Phase-IV, Kundli, Haryana.

# Editorial Board

**Priya Verma Gupta** MDS FPFA
Professor
Department of Pedodontics and Preventive Dentistry
Divya Jyoti College of Dental Sciences and Research
Modi Nagar, Niwari Road, Ghaziabad
Uttar Pradesh, India

**Gunjan Gupta** MDS
Assistant Professor
Department of Periodontics
Shree Bankey Bihari Dental College and Research Centre
Hapur Road, Ghaziabad
Uttar Pradesh, India

**Nishant Gupta** MDS
Assistant Professor
Department of Orthodontics and Dentofacial Orthopedics
Shree Bankey Bihari Dental College and Research Centre
Hapur Road, Ghaziabad
Uttar Pradesh, India

**Swati Tripathi** MDS
Associate Professor
Department of Pedodontics
Institute of Dental Sciences
Bareilly, Uttar Pradesh, India

# Preface

I am very pleased to introduce you to the first edition of Essential Quick Review; A series for final year undergraduate students.

The series will be available in eight subjects, i.e., Periodontics, Endodontics and Conservative Dentistry, Paedodontics, Prosthodontics, Oral Surgery, Oral Medicine and Radiology, Orthodontics and Public Health Dentistry covering essential parts of each subject. This book will not only help the student to attain the knowledge, but will also give an idea how to attempt a question during the examination, covering entire syllabus in a limited period of time.

It is a supplementary booklet for each subject that contains three sections, i.e., definitions, classifications and viva voce covering the entire syllabus enabling the student to undergo a quick revision. The language used is very simple for better understanding.

The study material provided in this book is an attempt to provide an additional help to students for easy retention and reproduction of subject in the examination. This book is in no way a replacement to standard text book.

I thank all my subject matter experts for their valued suggestions and contributions. A very special word of thanks to my family for being the source of constant encouragement.

I profusely thank Shri Jitendar P Vij (CEO), Mr Ankit Vij (Group President), and production team of M/S Jaypee Brothers Medical Publishers (P) Ltd, New Delhi for their enthusiasm and constant efforts in bringing out this book.

**Priya Verma Gupta**

# Contents

# Definitions

**Aberrancy**

It is defined as that situation in which a tissue develops at a site where it is not normally found.

**Aberration**

It is a variation from the normal form or course.

**Abfraction**

Loss of tooth surface at the cervical areas of teeth, caused by tensile and compressive forces during tooth flexure; cervical erosive lesions that can not be attributed to any particular cause.

**Ablation**

It is removal of a part by excision or amputation.

**Abnormal**

It is not normal, deviating in some form from the usual structure, position or state.

**Abocclusion**

It is a condition where the maxillary and mandibular teeth are not in contact.

**Abrasion**

It is the wearing away of a structure or substance by mechanical means such as scrubbing or grinding.

**Abrasive**

It is a substance which contains an abrasive which tends to erode the surface.

**Abscess**

An abscess is a localised collection of pus surrounded by an area of inflamed tissue in which hyperemia and infiltration of leukocytes is marked.

**Acantholysis**

The pathological separation of epidermal or epithelial cells by breakdown of desmosomes in stratum spinosum (seen in pemphigus).

**Acanthosis**

This condition is characterised by widening and thickening of stratum spinosum.

**Acquired**

Relating to something not of genetic origin but resulting from outside influence.

**Acrocephalic**

A highly arched or pointed skull.

**Actinic cheilitis**

When this atrophic tissue abrades to ulcer, it is called as actinic cheilitis.

**Actinic elastosis**

A lesion on the labial mucosa exposed to sun. A white area of atrophic epithelium develops with underlying scarring of the lamina propria.

**Actinic keratosis**

A premalignant squamous cell lesion resulting from long-term exposure to solar radiation and may be found on the vermilion border of lip as well as other sun exposed skin surfaces.

**Acute**

Having severe symptoms and a short course.

**Adduction**

Drawing in towards the center or to median line, as opposed to abduction.

**Adenomatosis oris**

The swelling of the mucous glands of the lips with no inflammation or secretion.

**Adrenodontia**

A morphological indication of over activity of adrenal glands characterised by large pointed canines and teeth with occlusal surfaces showing brown discoloration.

**Aerodontia**

That branch of dentistry concerned with the care and treatment of dental conditions caused by high altitude flying.

**Afferent nerve**

It refers to any nerve transmitting impulse from the periphery to the center.

**Ageusia**

Loss or absence of sense of taste.

**Aglossostomia**

Congenital absence of the tongue and of mouth opening.

**Agranulocytosis**

A marked decrease in the number of granulocytes, particularly neutrophils.

**Allelograft**

A graft using material not derived from a donor or from animal sources, e.g.,, synthetic resins, stainless steel alloy.

**Allergen**

A substance capable of inducing hypersensitivity or an allergic reaction.

**Allergy**

Hypersensitivity to any normally harmless substance resulting in an exaggerated or abnormal reaction.

**Allograft**

A graft derived from a donor of the same species but genetically dissimilar.

**Amalgam tattoo**

Oral soft tissue discolorations due to amalgam; most common pigmentation of the oral cavity.

**Amelogenesis**

The formation of the enamel portion of the tooth.

**Amniocentesis**

The diagnostic procedure in which a small amount of amniotic fluid is withdrawn from amniotic sac, a membrane surrounding the fetus in uterus, to detect fetal defects.

**Anachoresis**

If the bacteria circulating in the bloodstream settle in areas of inflammation or of lowered resistance in the pulp and produce pulpitis, abscess or necrosis, the phenomenon is referred to as anachoresis.

**Analgesia**

Relief from pain or insensitivity to pain.

**Analogous**

Having similar properties.

**Anaphylaxis**

An antigen-antibody reaction produced by the parenteral injection of an antigen causing hypersensitivity.

**Anaplasia**

The reversion of the same type of cells from a more highly differentiated to a less highly differentiated type.

**Anastomosis**

Communication between two vessels.

**Anemia**

An abnormal reduction in the number of circulating red blood cells, the quantity of hemoglobin and the volume of packed red cells in a given unit of blood.

**Anesthesia**

General loss of all sensations or feelings.

**Angioma**

A tumor made up of blood or lymph vessels.

**Ankyloglossia**

The extensive adhesion of the tongue to the floor of the mouth or the lingual aspect of the anterior portion of the mandible due to the presence of a short lingual frenum.

**Anomalad**

A malformation together with its subsequently derived structural changes; the primary defect setting off a series of secondary or even tertiary events resulting in multiple anomalies

**Anomaly**

Deviation or irregularity as compared with the normal.

**Anorexia**

Lack of appetite.

**Anosmia**

Absence of sense of smell.

**Antagonist**

Any tissue that acts against or in opposition to another tissue.

**Antibiotics**

Substances produced by microorganisms which suppress the growth or kill other microorganisms at a very low concentration.

**Antibody**

Any one of the class of substances produced in the body as a reaction to a specific antigen and with which, it reacts in some observable way to produce a specific effect such as inactivation, agglutination, and/or flocculation.

**Antidote**

An agent used to counteract or prevent the action of poisons.

**Antigen**

Any substance that when introduced into the body, excites the formation of specific antibodies.

**Apertognathia (open bite)**

A condition in which the anterior or the posterior teeth of the mandible can not be brought into occlusion with antagonist teeth of maxilla.

**Aplasia**

Absence of an organ or organ's part due to failure of development of the embryonic tissue of origin.

**Aponeurosis**

These are collagenous sheets or ribbons that resemble flat, broad tendons. It may cover the surface of the muscle and assist in attaching superficial muscles or separate the structures.

**Arteriosclerosis**

A condition characterised by loss of elasticity and thickening of artery walls.

**Atresia**

Congenital occlusion or absence of one or two major salivary gland ducts.

**Atrophy**

Reduction in size of tissue or of an organ due to decrease in the size or number of its constituent cells.

**Attrition**

Physiologic wearing away of tooth material as a result of tooth to tooth contact.

**Atypical**

Irregular, not confirmable to the type.

**Auscultation**

Listening to the sound produced within the body with the help of a stethoscope.

**Autoantibody**

An antibody that reacts against an antigenic constituent of the person's own tissues.

**Autogenous**

It is produced within the body itself. It is self-generated.

**Autograft**

It is a graft taken from one of the patient's body and transplanted to another part in the same individual.

**Autoimmune disease**

A disease characterised by tissue injury caused by a humoral or cell-mediated immune response against constituents of the body's own tissues.

**Autoimmunity**

Immune-mediated destruction of the body's own cells and tissues; immunity against self.

**Autoinoculation**

The process to inoculate with a pathogen such as a virus from one's own body.

**Autosomes**

The non-sex chromosomes that are identical for men and women.

**Bacteremia**

It refers to the circulation of bacteria in the blood.

**Bacteria**

These are microscopic unicellular vegetative organisms having a single chromosome, no nuclear envelope and a rigid cell wall. They may be seen as rods, cocci or filaments and divide by binary fission.

**Bacteriostatic**

It is any agent that inhibits the growth and multiplication of bacteria.

**Baelz's disease**

It is a disease characterised by the presence of painless papules on the labial mucous membrane (Cheilitis glandularis superficial suppurative type).

**Ballooning degeneration**

It is characterised by the isolation of a cell from its neighbors, especially in the lower layers of the epidermis, the withdrawing of its prickles after intra-cytoplasmic edema and vacuolization and the mitotic division of its nucleus so as to form multinucleated giant cells.

**Bay cyst**

Apical cyst which has a direct connection with apical foramen has been termed as 'bay cyst.'

**Bednar's aphthae**

Two ulcers appearing symmetrically one on either side of the midline of the hard palate in infants, thought to be caused by the nipple or by thumb sucking or sucking hard object.

**Benign**

Not malignant; favourable for recovery.

**Bicameral abscess**

It is an abscess which contains two chambers.

**Biopsy**

It is the gross and microscopic examination of tissue or cells removed from living patients for the purpose of diagnosis or prognosis of the disease or the confirmation of the normal condition.

**Blanching**

To take the color out of and make white.

**Bleb**

It is a bulla or other skin blister filled with blood or serous fluid.

**Blind abscess**

It is the one having no fistulous tracts.

**Blister**

It is a vesicle caused by localised accumulation of fluid beneath the skin.

**Blood**

Red fluid in the vessels of the circulating system which conveys oxygen and nutritive materials to the tissue and removes carbon dioxide and waste matter.

**Blood pressure**

Pressure exerted by the blood on the artery walls and is dependent on the force of heart action, the elasticity of the vessel walls, capillary and the volume and viscosity of blood.

**Blood transfusion**

The intravenous administration of blood to help replenish excess blood loss due to haemorrhage or otherwise, is known as blood transfusion.

**Boil**

It is a localised skin abscess usually at the site of a hair follicle.

**Bosselated**

Having a knob like protrusion or bosses.

**Bowen's disease**

It is a localised intra-epidermoid carcinoma that may progress to invasive carcinoma over many years.

**Bradycardia**

An abnormal slowness of the heart and pulse rate.

**Bradyglossia**

Abnormal slowness of speech, due to difficulty in tongue movements.

**Bradypnea**

Abnormal slowness of respiration.

**Bruise**

It is a superficial injury, caused by a blow with no laceration but with discoloration of the skin and subcutaneous tissue produced by an accumulation of blood.

**Bruxism**

It can be defined as the involuntary, unconscious, and excessive grinding, tapping or clenching of teeth or it is defined as non-functional grinding or gnashing of the teeth, usually during sleep.

**Buccal bifurcation cyst**

A cyst of uncertain origin found primarily on the distal or facial aspect of a vital mandibular third molar, consisting of intensely inflamed connective tissue and epithelial lining.

**Bullae**

An elevated blister like lesion containing clear fluid and is bigger than 1 cm in diameter.

**Burn**

Injury resulting from the application of excessive heat, electric current, friction and caustics to skin or mucous membrane.

**Burrows**

Short, linear, straight or sinuous lines in the skin.

**Calcareous**

Relating to or containing calcium or calcium salts; chalky.

**Calcification**

It is the deposition of inorganic tissue of calcium salts causing hardening.

**Calcinosis**

It is a condition characterised by either localised or generalized deposition of calcium salts in nodules in the soft tissues.

**Callus**

The mesh of fibrous bony tissue surrounding and uniting the bone ends after fracture. It is later replaced by hard bone.

**Camper's line**

It is the line extending from the external auditory meatus to a point below the nasal point and is also called as facial line.

**Cancellous**

Having a lattice like spongy structure; particularly applied for bone tissue.

**Canker**

An ulceration especially of the mouth and lips, also called as aphthous stomatitis.

**Capillary**

These are one of the very fine thread like blood vessels connecting the veins and arteries.

**Capsule**

Compressed fibrous connective tissue around a benign neoplasm separating it from surrounding tissues.

**Carabelli's cusp**

It is an accessory lingual cusp located on mesiopalatine cusp of maxillary second primary molars and 1st, 2nd and 3rd permanent molars.

**Carbuncle**

It is a staphylococcal infection of the sweat glands or hair follicles causing inflammation of the surrounding subcutaneous tissue and discharging pus through several openings, finally sloughing away.

**Carcinogenesis/Oncogenesis/Tumorogenesis**

Induction of a tumor agent which can induce tumor. The tumor agents are called as carcinogens.

**Carcinoma**

A malignant growth made up of epithelial cells that are capable of infiltration and metastasis.

**Carcinoma in situ**

It is a histopathological diagnosis defined as a proliferation of basal epithelial cells from the basement membrane to the surface, with almost all of the cells manifesting cytologic atypia. Immediate maturation into a superficial keratin layer is possible, but no invasion into the underlying connective tissues can be seen.

**Carcinosarcoma**

It is a mixed tumor containing characteristics of both carcinoma and sarcoma.

**Caries**

Irreversible microbial disease of the calcified tissues of the teeth, characterized by demineralization of inorganic portion and destruction of the organic substance of the tooth surface, which often leads to cavitation.

**Cariology**

The scientific study of dental caries, its causes, prevention and treatment.

**Carrier**

The individual who continues to harbor infectious agent either following recovery from the illness it induced.

**Cartilage**

It is a form of elastic, nonvascular connective tissue attached to articular bone surfaces and also forming some parts of the skeleton.

**Catabolism**

Process of breakdown of complex compounds by the body.

**Catarrh**

It is the inflammation of the mucous membranes, especially those of nose and throat, with discharge of mucus.

**Causalgia**

Burning sensation arising after trauma to a sensory nerve.

**Cell**

It is one of the minute masses of protoplasm, containing a nucleus which forms the basis of all animal and plant structure.

**Cell mediated immunity**

The type of immunity in which the predominant role is played by T-lymphocytes.

**Cellulitis**

A non-suppurative inflammation of the subcutaneous tissue extending along the connective tissue planes and across the intercellular spaces.

**Cementicle**

It is a small calcareous body developing in the periodontal membrane.

**Central**

In oral pathology, it is the lesion occurring within bone.

**Centromere**

The constricted portion of the chromosome that divides the short arms from the long arms.

**Cheesy**

Lesion's texture is similar to curd or cheese.

**Cheilitis**

Inflammation of lip.

**Chemoprophylaxis**

Use of chemical drugs in the prevention of disease.

**Chemotaxis**

Taxis or movement in response to chemical stimulation.

**Chemotherapy**

It is the treatment of a disease by chemicals which affect pathogenic organisms without harming the patient or it is the treatment of malignant neoplasia by chemical means.

**Chief complaint**

It is the patient's response to the dentist's question.

**Chills**

It is cold sensation with shivering, often characteristic of onset of fever.

**Chloroma**

It is a condition characterised by multiple myeloid tumors of greenish color, affecting particularly the face and skull, and associated with blood picture of leukemia.

**Chondromalacia**

A condition characterised by abnormal softness of the cartilage.

**Choriostoma**

The excessive amount of normal tissue that is present in abnormal location.

**Chromatin**

A general term used to refer to the material (DNA) that forms the chromosomes.

**Chronic**

Persisting over a long time; when applied to a disease, chronic means that there has been little change or extremely slow progression over a long period.

**Ciliated**

Having hair like processes or fringe of hair.

**Circulation**

It is the movement or flow in a circle, retracing its course repeatedly, applied especially to the flow of blood through the body.

**Cleft lip**

A birth defect that results in a unilateral or bilateral opening in the upper lip between the mouth and the nose.

**Cleft palate**

A birth defect characterised by an opening in the roof of the mouth caused by lack of tissue development.

**Coagulation**

When blood is shed, it loses its fluidity in few minutes and sets into a semisolid jelly. This is called as coagulation or clotting.

**Coalesce**

It is a term used to denote to fusion or union of separated parts.

**Coarctation**

Narrowing or constriction, applied especially to blood vessels.

**Col**

A depression in an interdental papilla between the two peaks, one on each side of the contact area.

**Cold abscess**

A slow developing tuberculous abscess generally about a bone or joint and with little inflammation.

**Collar stud abscess**

A superficial abscess connected by a sinus tract to a larger deep abscess.

**Coma**

A state of complete unconsciousness from which a patient can not be aroused, even by determined external stimulation.

**Commensal**

It is an organism that lives on or within another organism, to its own advantage and without being detrimental to the host.

**Commissure**

It is the point of union between similar parts or bodies.

**Complement system**

This consists of a group of serum proteins which by series of reactions produce and release by products whose functions are to initiate an inflammatory reaction, to regulate and enhance phagocytic function and attack the bacterial cell membrane.

**Concrescence**

It is a form of fusion that occurs after the root and other major parts of the involved teeth are formed or when the roots of two or more teeth are united by cementum, below the cementoenamel junction.

**Concretion**

It refers to any hardened or solidified mass in the tissue.

**Congenital**

Present at or before birth but not necessarily inherited.

**Consanguinity**

Blood relationship. In genetics, the term is generally used to describe marriages among close relatives.

**Corrugated**

Having a surface that appears wrinkled.

**Counter irritation**

Deliberate production of superficial irritation in order to mask or relieve an existing irritation or pain.

**Craniomalacia**

It refers to a condition characterised by softness of bones of the skull, usually seen in infants.

**Crater**

It is a localised depression, usually circular, with raised edge or rim.

**Crepitations**

Crackling noise occurring in the joint when affected by certain disease.

**Crust**

Dry products of exudation from lesions occurring on skin and lips.

**Cryosurgery**

The use of extreme cold produced by liquid nitrogen (or argon gas) for surgical destruction of abnormal tissue.

**Cryotherapy**

Treatment of disease with general or local use of low temperature.

**Cryptogenic leukoplakia**

In a small proportion of cases of leukoplakia, no underlying cause has been found. Such lesions are termed as idiopathic or cryptogenic leukoplakia.

**Culture**

It is the growth of microorganisms in an artificial medium.

**Curettage**

Removal of foreign matter from the walls of a bony cavity or from the root surface.

**Cyanosis**

The bluish discoloration of the skin and mucous membranes, often due to deficient oxygenation of the blood.

**Cyst**

Cyst is a pathological cavity which may or may not be lined by epithelium and consists of fluid, semi-fluid or gaseous content but not by accumulation of pus and is surrounded by connective tissue capsule. True cyst is a pathologic cavity always lined by epithelium.

**Cytology**

Scientific study of cell.

**Cytopathic**

- Pertaining to or characterised by pathologic changes in cells.

**Debridment**

It is the removal of dead tissue and foreign matter from a wound.

**Degeneration**

The gradual deterioration of tissue involving chemical changes along with loss of function.

**Dens evaginatus**

Dens evaginatus is a developmental condition that appears clinically as an accessory cusp or globules of enamel on occlusal surface between buccal and lingual cusp of premolars.

**Dens in dente (Dens invaginatus)**

Developmental variation which is thought to arise as a result of invagination in the surface of tooth crown before calcification has occured.

**Dental fluorosis**

A condition of enamel hypoplasia characterised by white chalky spots or brown staining and pitting of teeth due to an increased level of fluoride; affecting enamel matrix formation and calcification by impairment of ameloblastic function.

**Dental kinesiology**

It is the study of motion and function of jaws and oral musculature; the accompanying neurological, vascular and other supporting system network and the impact of those muscle functions and neurological dynamics have on dental and systemic health.

**Dentigerous cyst**

An odontogenic cyst that surrounds the crown of an impacted tooth; caused by fluid accumulation between the reduced enamel epithelium and enamel surface.

**Dentistry**

It is a branch of medicine concerned with oral and dental diseases, their prevention, treatment and oral prosthesis.

**Dentoalveolar abscess**

An abscess that forms at the end of the tooth root.

**Deoxyribonucleic acid (DNA)**

A substance composed of a double chain of polynucleotide; both chains coiled around a central axis to form a double helix. DNA is the basic genetic code or template for amino acid formation.

**Dermoid cyst**

A cyst of midline of the upper neck or the anterior floor of the mouth of young patients, derived from remnants of embryonic skin; consisting of a lumen lined by a keratinizing stratified squamous epithelium and containing one or more skin appendages such as hair, sweat or sebaceous glands.

**Desmosomes**

The structures forming the site of contact between adjacent cells, especially epithelial cells.

**Desquamation**

It refers to the peeling off of the outer layer of epithelium.

**Developmental anomalies**

Malformation or defects resulting from disturbance of growth and development are known as developmental anomalies.

**Diagnosis**

It is the determination of the nature or cause of the disease.

**Differential diagnosis**

The list of similar clinical picture, according to probable identity of condition at hand, is the differential diagnosis.

**Diffuse**

It is to describe of a lesion; if borders of the lesion are not well defined and it is not possible to detect the exact parameters of the lesion.

**Dilacerations**

Angulations or sharp bends or curves in the root and crown of the teeth.

**Dimorphic anemia**

It is a condition in which iron deficiency and folic acid deficiency anemia can occur concomitantly.

**Direct fracture**

Fracture that occurs at the site of blow.

**Discrete**

Composed of separate parts, not joined or blended.

**Disease**

It is the departure from the average anatomical structure or is an abnormal degree of failure of physiological function or some reduction in psychological efficiency, due to either adversity in the genetic endowment of the individual or misuse of his free will or to adverse factors in the environment in which he lives or some combination of these factors or it is defined as loss of ease.

**Disinfection**

The process by which pathogenic microorganisms are removed from the surface, without removing bacterial spores.

**Dislocation**

The displacement of any part from its normal position, especially in the cases of bones and joints.

**Distomolar**

Found in the molar region frequently located distal to 3rd molar.

**Diverticuli**

They are small pouches or out pocket of the ductal system of one of the major salivary glands.

**DLE (discoid lupus erythematous)**

It is a circumscribed slightly elevated white patch, usually surrounded by a red telangiectic halo.

**Dominant**

In genetics, a trait or characteristic that is manifested when it is carried by only one of a pair of homologous chromosomes.

**Dorsal**

Directed towards or situated on the back surface (opposite of ventral).

**Dose**

It is one measured portion of any medicine which is to be taken one at a time.

**Drainage**

It is the gradual removal of fluid from a cavity or wound.

**Dressing**

It is a medicament used to promote wound healing or as a covering for a wound, used for protection or to assist healing.

**Drug**

Any medicinal substance.

**Drug abuse/misuse**

It is the improper or excessive use of therapeutic drugs even in the absence of addiction.

**Drug addiction**

It is state of periodic or chronic intoxication produced by the repeated consumption of drug and is harmful to individual and to society.

**Drug dependence**

A state psychic and sometimes also physical resulting from the interaction between a living organism and a drug, characterised by behavioral and other response that always includes a compulsion to the drug on a continuous or periodic basis in order to experience its psychic effect and sometimes to avoid the discomfort of its absence.

**Drug habituation**

It is the condition resulting from repeated consumption of drug, in which there is psychological and emotional dependency on the drug.

**Dry abscess**

An abscess that disperses without bursting or coming to a head.

**Dysesthesia**

It refers to the impairment of feeling or sensations; a condition in which a normal stimulus produces disagreeable sensations.

**Dyskeratosis**

The condition an abnormal orientation in development of epithelial cells.

**Dyskinesia**

It is defined as an impairment of voluntary motions, causing movements that are incomplete or only partial.

**Dysodontiasis**

It refers to the painful, difficult or delayed eruption of the teeth.

**Dysostosis**

It refers to the congenital defective bone formation.

**Dysphagia**

Difficulty in swallowing.

**Dysplasia**

It refers to the abnormal growth or formation.

**Dyspnea**

Shortness of breath.

**Dystrophic calcification**

Pathologic calcification that occurs in degenerating and dead tissue.

**Ecchymosis**

It refers to the diffuse extravasation of blood into the tissues. Larger purpuric lesions are called as ecchymoses.

**Ectoderm**

The outermost layer of the three primary germ layers of the embryo, which gives rise to the epidermis, the external sense organs, oral and anal mucous membranes.

**Edema**

It is accumulation of excess fluid in the intercellular tissue spaces or body cavities.

**Electrocautery(Electrocauterization)**

A small probe with low voltage current is used to burn or destroy the unwanted or harmful tissue. It can also be used to burn and seal blood vessel to reduce or stop bleeding during surgery or after injury

**Electrodesiccation**

The deeply penetrating tissue dehydration caused by the insertion of electrodes into the tissue.

**Embedded teeth**

Teeth which are unerupted usually due to lack of eruptive forces.

**Embolism**

The sudden blockage of blood vessels by a clot or other obstruction within the blood stream, causing decreased or failure of circulation.

**Embryonic**

Pertaining to the earliest developmental stage of of an organism.

**Emigration**

The passage of leukocytes through walls of small blood vessels.

**Empirical therapy**

A reasonable, pregmatic approach to begin antibiotic therapy before result of cultural investigations with an effort to direct treatment towards organisms which are most likely to have caused that infection.

**Empyema**

It is the accumulation of pus in a body cavity or a hollow organ.

**Enamel pearls, nodules, or droplets**

Small nodules of enamel usually about 1–2 mm in diameter that form on the root end or at the bifurcation of multi-rooted teeth.

**Enanthema**

It is an eruption occurring on a mucous surface or on any other surface within the body as opposed to exanthema.

**Endemic**

Prevalent in a particular region.

**Endodermal**

Pertaining to the innermost of the three primitive germ layers of an embryo. Endodermal structures include the epithelium pharynx, respiratory tract (except the nose) and digestive tract.

**Endosteal**

It is within the bone.

**Endothelium**

It refers to the membrane lining the heart and blood vessels.

**Endotoxin**

These are heat stable phospholipid-polysaccharide-protein complex present as a structural part of the cell of many

Gram Negative bacterias and released by disintegration of the cells.

**Engorgement**

It refers to the excess of blood in any part of the body. It is the localised congestion or distension.

**Enostosis**

A localised morbid bone growth arising within the bone cavity.

**Enucleate**

The word enucleate means to remove an organ or part, circumscribed or space filling lesion entirely, from its outer sheath or covering.

**Epidemic**

Affecting large number of people within an area or region.

**Epidemiology**

It is that branch of science concerned with the study of a disease or condition through its frequency and distribution.

**Epithelium**

It is a thin cellular layer covering or lining the organs and tissues of the body.

**Eponym**

The name of an organ, syndrome, disease, etc. that contains or is derived from a proper name.

**Epulis**

Any tumor of the gums; particularly fibrous or a giant cell tumor.

**Erosion (teeth)**

It is loss of tooth substance due to chemical process that does not involve bacterial activity.

**Erosion**

It is a shallow crater in the epithelial surface that appears on clinical examination as a very shallow erythematous area with only superficial changes or a moist red lesion often caused by rupture in vesicles and bullae as well as trauma.

**Eruption**

The act of appearing or pushing through, as of teeth coming through the gums or a visible skin lesion occurring in disease.

**Erythema**

It is the redness in the skin either diffuse or patchy, caused by congestion of the subcutaneous capillaries.

**Erythematous**

It characterised by redness of the tissue due to engorgement of the capillaries in affected region.

**Erythrocyte**

A type of red cell found in blood which carries oxygen and is produced by the bone marrow.

**Erythrodontia**

There is deposition of porphyrins in dentin and to a lesser extent in the enamel which imparts red or brown color to the deciduous and permanent teeth.

**Erythroplakia**

The term is applied to any area of reddened velvety textured mucosa that is difficult to be diagnosed on the basis of clinical and histopathological examination as a cause of inflammation or any other disease process.

**Erythroplasia**

These are painless erythematous eruptions, papular or macular in nature, affecting the mucous membrane.

**Erythroplastic**

It is characterised by a reddish appearance. This term implies abnormal tissue proliferation in the reddish area.

**Eschar**

It is a dry slough caused by burning or contact with a corrosive agent.

**Etiology**

The study or theory of the factors that cause disease.

**Eversion**

A turning outward or a state being turned outwards.

**Exacerbation**

It refers to an increase in the severity of a disease or any symptoms.

**Examination**

It refers to investigations carried out for diagnostic purpose.

**Exanthema**

It is an eruptive fever.

**Excoriation**

It is the superficial loss of surface skin or a graze.

**Excrescence**

It refers to an abnormal growth protruding from body or plant.

**Excursion**

It refers to any movement of a movable part from a resting position during the performance of some functions.

**Exfoliation**

It is the peeling off in layers or in scales.

**Exophthalmos**

It refers to the abnormal protrusion of the eyeball.

**Exophytic**

It refers to a word relating to something growing outwards, used for tumor projecting above the normal surface contours.

**Exostosis**

It is a bony swelling developing on the bone surface or root of tooth.

**Exotoxin**

It refers to a toxic secretion of bacterial cells which cause damage in sites distant from the focus of infections. These are heat labile proteins which are secreted by certain bacteria and diffuse readily into surrounding tissue.

**Expansile**

Capable of being extended or expanded.

**Expressivity**

In genetics, the degree of clinical manifestation of a trait or characteristic.

**Extravasation**

It is the escape of fluid from vessels into the surrounding tissue.

**Extrinsic**

Having its origin outside and separated from a body, organ or part.

**Exudate**

The matter that passes out into adjacent tissues through vessel walls in inflammation.

**Facet**

It is a small abraded area on a bone or on tooth surface.

**Facies**

The appearance of the face.

**Factitial injuries**

These are accidentally self-induced injuries on the basis of habits with frequent psychological backgrounds.

**Familial**

Relating to a family, or affecting several of its members.

**Fascia**

It is the layer of areolar tissue beneath the skin or investing the muscles, nerves and other organs.

**Favorable fracture**

If the fracture line runs in such a manner that the associated muscle tends to hold the fragments together, the fracture is described as favorable.

**Fenestrate**

To pierce with one or more holes, sometimes used on the walls of bony defect in an attempt to stimulate repair.

**Fenestration**

It refers to a surgical procedure by which one or more holes are pierced in hard tissue.

**Fever**

It refers to an abnormal increase in body temperature.

**Fibro-cemento-osseous lesions**

It is a skeletal disorder in which bone is replaced by fibrous tissue which in turn is replaced by mineralized tissue.

**Fibrosis**

An abnormal formation of fibrous tissue.

**Final diagnosis**

It is statement with which precise diagnosis has been made on the basis of all required observation, identification of definitive symptoms, histopathological report and patient response to therapy.

**Fissure**

It is a linear often crusted, tender, painful defect in continuity of the skin, occurring usually at the mucocutaneous junctions and at sites where there is considerable elasticity of the skin.

**Fistula**

It is communicating tract between two epithelial surfaces which is lined by granulation tissue which is subsequently epithelialized.

**Fluctuant**

A wave-like motion felt on palpating a cavity with non-rigid walls, especially one containing fluid.

**Fluoride mottling**

A condition of enamel hypoplasia characterised by white chalky spots or brown staining and pitting of teeth due to an increased level of fluoride affecting enamel matrix formation and calcification by impairment of ameloblastic function.

**Focal infection**

It refers to metastasis from the focus of infection of organisms or their products that are capable of injuring tissue.

**Focal osteitis**

A condition sometimes occurring after tooth extraction, particularly after traumatic extraction, resulting in a dry appearance of the exposed bone in the socket, due to disintegration or loss of the blood clot.

**Focus of infection**

It refers to a circumscribed area of tissue, which is infected with exogenous pathogenic microorganisms and which is usually located near a mucous or cutaneous surface.

**Foramen**

A small hole in a bone through which passes either blood vessels or nerves or both.

**Foreign body granuloma**

A reaction to foreign materials that are too large to be ingested by either microphages (PMN s) or macrophages.

**Frenal tag**

A redundant piece of mucosal tissue that projects from the maxillary labial frenum.

**Fulguration**

It refers to the superficial tissue dehydration produced by a surgical electrode held slightly away from the tissue, causing sparking.

**Fusion**

It is also called as synodontia. It represents the embryonic union of normally separated tooth germs.

**Galvanism**

The production of an electric current caused when two dissimilar metals used as restorations in the mouth come into contact, this can cause discomfort and even pain.

**Gangrene**

It is the necrosis of tissue due to failure of the arterial blood supply caused by injury or disease.

**Gelation**

The process of change of a colloid from a sol to a gel.

**Gemination**

It refers to the process whereby single tooth germ invaginates resulting in incomplete formation of two teeth that may appear as a bifid crown on a single root.

**Genetic heterogeneity**

Having more than one inheritance pattern.

**Gerodontia**

It is that branch of dentistry which deals with the care of old people.

**Ghost teeth**

A developmental disturbance of several adjacent teeth in which the enamel and dentin are thin and irregular and fail to adequately mineralize; surrounding soft tissue is hyperplastic and contains focal accumulations of spherical calcifications and odontogenic rests.

**Gingivosis**

It refers to any degenerative condition affecting the gingiva.

**Gland**

An organ that produces secretions.

**Glossodynia**

It refers to the burning or painful condition of the tongue.

**Gomphosis**

It is the firm attachment of two bones without a movable joint.

**Gorham's disease**

In this condition a large portion of bone disappears without any apparent cause.

**Granulation tissue**

It is the reparative tissue that is formed on the surface of wound having pink, soft, granular appearance showing histologically new small blood vessel and fibroblasts.

**Granuloma**

A tumor composed of granulation tissue.

**Granulomatosis**

It refers to the development of multiple granuloma.

**Green stick bone fracture**

It is a fracture in which one side of bone is broken and the other side is bent but intact.

**Ground glass**

Fine radiopaque spots in radiolucent background.

**Gustatory**

The sense of taste or the act of tasting.

**Habit**

It is a tendency towards an act or an act that has become a repeated performance, relatively fixed, constant, easy to perform and almost automatic.

**Hamartomas**

It is a tumor like malformation of oral tissues, developmental in origin with tissue being native to the site.

**Healing**

It is repair and replacement of dead or damaged cells by healthy cells.

**Hematoma**

It is large clot resulting from blood released into the tissue from a ruptured or injured blood vessel.

**Hemidesmosome**

It refers to a structure found on the basal surface of an epithelial cell, the attachment site between the cell and the underlying membrane.

**Hemoglobinopathies**

These are a group of hereditary disorders characterised by the presence of structurally abnormal hemoglobin.

**Hemoptysis**

The presence of blood in the sputum caused by bleeding in the upper respiratory tract or the lungs.

**Haemorrhage**

It refers to the internal or external loss of blood due to injury or other damage to blood vessels.

**Hereditary disease**

They are apparent at birth but some may not become evident for years.

**Heredity**

It refers to the transmission of a characteristic from parent to child or to later generation.

**Heterotrophic**

It is a term used relating to organisms which require a complex source of carbon for nourishment and growth.

**Histology**

It refers to the study of the anatomy and physiology of tissue and cells using microscopic technique.

**Holistic**

It refers to an approach to treatment that takes into consideration the whole person, not just the disease or condition.

**Homologous**

Having the same or corresponding structure or position but not necessary similar in function.

**Horner's teeth**

Incisor teeth with horizontal grooves caused by enamel deficiency.

**Hydrocyst**

It refers to a cyst whose contents are watery in nature.

**Hydropic degeneration**

It refers to replacement of the nuclei of stratum basal by clear space due to edema and degeneration of cells.

**Hydrostomia**

It refers to a condition characterised by constant dribbling from the mouth.

**Hygroma**

It refers to a swelling caused by fluid surrounding an inflamed bursa, or distending a sac or cyst.

**Hyperplasia**

It refers to the enlargement caused by increase in number of cells.

**Hypertension**

Exceptionally high tension especially abnormally high blood pressure.

**Hypertrophy**

It refers to the enlargement caused by an increase in size of cells.

**Hypnosis**

It refers to a sleep or a trance state, especially one induced artificially by verbal suggestions or concentration upon some object.

**Hypodontia**

It refers to the absence of one or more teeth.

**Hypoplasia**

It is the failure of full development of an organ or tissue.

**Hypsodont**

Having teeth with long crowns and short roots seen in herbivorous animals.

**Iatrogenic diseases**

These are the diseases produced by the action of a doctor or due to medical treatment.

**Idiopathic**

It is any spontaneous or primary disease with no apparent external cause.

**Idiosyncrasy**

It refers to a reaction to a particular drug in therapeutic doses in a manner not necessarily related to its pharmacological properties.

**Immunity**

It is the resistance exhibited by the host towards injury caused by microorganisms and their products.

**Impacted teeth**

They are those prevented from erupting by some physical barriers in the eruption path.

**Impermeable**

Not permitting passage especially of fluids.

**Implant**

The word implant means to insert into the body or to graft as in plastic surgery.

**Indentation**

It refers to the condition of being serrated or notched.

**Indirect fracture**

Fracture site distant from where the actual blow takes place, usually seen on contralateral side.

**Induced**

Brought on by an outside agent or is artificially produced.

**Induration**

It refers to the state of being hard or the process of becoming hard.

**Infarction**

It is a localised area of ischemic necrosis in an organ or tissue resulting from sudden reduction of either its arterial supply or venous drainage.

**Infection**

It is a clinicopathological entity-involving invasion of the body by pathologic microorganisms and the reaction of tissues to microorganism and their toxins.

**Inflammation**

It is the reaction of living tissue to injury.

**Inflammatory collateral cyst**

It is a cyst which arises in the periodontium of an erupted tooth as a result of inflammatory process in the periodontal pocket.

**Inflation**

It refers to the distension with gas especially air.

**Inostosis**

It refers to the process by which bony tissue is reformed to replace tissue that has been destroyed.

**Insidious**

Unperceived coming on gradually and stealthily.

**Inspection**

It refers to an examination of the affected part of the body.

**Intermittent**

Occurring at intervals with periods of cessation.

**Internal derangement**

Disruption within the internal aspects of TMJ in which there is a displacement of disc from its normal functional relationship with the mandibular condyle and the articular portion of the temporal bone.

**Intubation**

It refers to the introduction of a tube through the mouth or the nose to allow air, gas or vapor to pass into the lungs.

**In vitro**

Within glass referring to observations made in a test tube or culture dish as opposed to in vivo.

**In vivo**

Within a living organism.

**Involucrum**

Small section of necrotic bone may be completely lysed, while a large one may get localised, and get separated and form shell of new bone called involucrum.

**Iontophoresis**

The therapeutic treatment by electrical introduction of ions into the body tissue.

**Ischemia**

The deficiency in the blood supply to a part or an organ which may be due to constriction, contraction or blocking of the arteries.

**Isograft**

A graft derived from one member of a pair of monozygotic twins and transplanted to the other.

**Jaw winking**

A movement of the lower jaw causing an involuntary movement of the eyelids.

**Joint**

The place of connection between two bones, allowing of more or less movement on articulation.

**Keloid**

A fibrous hyperplastic scar growth on the skin.

**Kernicterus**

Staining of brain tissue caused by accumulation of unconjugated bilirubin in the brain.

**Knitting**

The process of repair of a bone fracture.

**Lain's disease**

Burning of the tongue and the soft tissue of the mouth due to electrogalvanism caused by the use of dissimilar metals in dental restoration.

**Lancinating**

It is the term used to describe shooting, tearing or sharply cutting type of pain.

**Lesion**

A wound or injury or a patch of disease on the skin. A morbid change in tissue function.

**Leukoplakia**

A white patch or plaque, usually more than 5 mm, that cannot be scraped off and cannot be characterised clinically or pathologically as any other disease.

**Lichen planus**

Relatively common dermatitis occurs on skin and oral mucous membranes. It has a lace-like pattern which resemebles the one formed by algal and fungal colonies on the surfaces of rocks in nature.

**Lipomatosis**

It refers to excessive localised accumulation of fats in the tissues.

**Ludwig's angina**

This condition may be defined as an overwhelming rapidly spreading septic cellulitis involving submandibular, submental and sublingual space bilaterally.

**Lymph**

The clear fluid found in the lymphatics vessels.

**Lymphadenitis**

The inflammation of the lymph nodes.

**Maceration**

The softening of a substance by soaking in a liquid.

**Macule**

Well-circumscribed flat lesion that is noticeable due to the change from the normal skin color to red may be due to inflammation or pigmented due to presence of melanin hemosiderin or other drugs.

**Malocclusion**

Any deviation from the normal occlusion of the teeth resulting in impaired functions.

**Marrow**

The soft tissue canal and interstices of bones.

**Marsupialization**

An operation for the evacuation of a cyst and the suturing of its walls to the edges of the wound.

**Medicine**

The study and treatment of diseases especially treatment without recourse to surgery or any drug used for the treatment of the disease.

**Mesiodens**

A supernumerary tooth located at or near the midline in the incisal region of maxilla between the central incisors.

**Metabolism**

The physical and chemical changes in the tissue by which a living body is maintained and its energy is generated.

**Metaplasia**

It is a reversible change in which one adult cell type is replaced by another adult cell type.

**Metastasis**

It is defined as spread of tumor by invasion in such a way that discontinuous secondary tumor mass/masses arc formed at the site of lodgment.

**Mitosis**

It is the indirect division of cells, a typical method of cell reproduction.

**Mucocele**

It is a term used to describe swelling caused by pooling of saliva at the site of injured minor salivary gland.

**Mucus plug**

These are incompletely mineralized sialoliths.

**Muscle**

It is a contractile organ by means of which movement is produced in an animal organism.

**Muscle spasm**

A sudden involuntary contraction of the muscle or group of muscles attended by pain and interference with function.

**Myofacial pain Dysfunction Syndrome**

MPDS is a pain disorder in which unilateral pain is referred from the trigger points in myofacial structures, to the muscles of the head and neck.

**Narcosis**

A state of profound unconsciousness or stupor produced by drugs.

**Natal teeth**

These are teeth which are observed in the oral cavities at birth.

**Nausea**

A feeling of sickness or a tendency to vomit.

**Necrosis**

It is the sum of the morphologic changes that follow cell death in a living tissue or organs.

**Neonatal teeth**

These are teeth which erupt during the first 30 days of life.

**Neoplasia**

It is an abnormal mass of tissue, the growth of which exceeds and is un-coordinate with that of normal tissue and persists in the same excessive manner after cessation of stimuli which evoked the change.

**Neurotropic**

Attracted to or having an affinity for nervous tissue.

**Nevus**

It is circumscribed, small, elevated, flat and pigmented lesion of skin or oral mucosa that is congenital in origin.

**Nociceptive**

Relating to any pain producing stimulus, or to pain receptor nerves.

**Nodules**

This lesion is present deep in the dermis and epidermis and can be moved easily over them.

**Nosology**

It refers to the science of classification of disease.

**Numbness**

Pathological (or which may be deliberately induced as in cases of local anesthesia) partial or total loss of sensation.

**Nutrition**

The process by which food is assimilated.

**Ointment**

A fatty semisolid substance used as a base for local medicaments for external application.

**Oligodontia**

It is agenesis of a few numbers of teeth.

**Oncology**

The study of neoplasm.

**Operation**

Anything performed, especially any procedure by a surgeon, either with instruments or by hand.

**Oral medicine**

It is that area of dental practice which deals with diagnosis and treatment of oral disease by non-surgical means, which may be localised in the oral cavity or which may be oral manifestation of systemic disease and those phases of dental practice concerned with diagnosis and treatment of medically compromised patients.

**Oral submucus fibrosis**

An insidious chronic disease affecting any part of the oral cavity and sometimes the pharynx, proceeded by and/or associated with vesicle formation, it is always associated with juxtaepithelial inflammatory reaction followed by fibro-elastic changes of the lamina propria, with epithelial atrophy leading to stiffness of the oral mucosa and causing trismus and inability to eat.

**Organ**

Any separate part of the body having a specific function.

**Organism**

Any individual plant or animal or an organized body of living cells.

**Oroantral opening**

The accidental opening in the floor of maxillary sinus during dental extraction is called as oroantral opening.

**Orofacial clefts**

They are congenital deformities, which manifest at birth. Any disturbance during the embryological formation and development and growth of orofacial region will result in the formation of orofacial clefts.

**Osteomyelitis**

It is an inflammation of bone marrow that produce clinically apparent pus and secondarily affect the calcified component or it is an infection of bone that involves all three components: periosteum, cortex and marrow. It may defined as an inflammatory condition of the bone that begins as an infection of medullary cavity and the haversian system which extends to involve the periosteum of the affected area.

**Pain**

The distressing or unpleasant sensation transmitted by a sensory nerve usually indicative of injury or of disease.

**Palliation**

The act of alleviating or affording relief without curing.

**Palpation**

It refers to feeling of the affected part by hand.

**Papules**

These are solid lesions raised above the skin surface that are smaller than 1 cm in diameter.

**Parageusia**

An unpleasant taste in the mouth.

**Parakeratosis**

Any abnormality of the stratum corneum of the epidermis, which may be associated with inflammation of the prickle cell layers causing defective formation of keratin and characterised by the persistence of nuclei.

**Paralysis**

It is the loss or impairment of muscle function or sensation due to nerve injury or destruction of neurons.

**Paramolar**

It is a supernumerary molar usually small and rudimentary which is situated buccally or lingually to one of maxillary molars or interproximally between 1st, 2nd and 3rd maxillary molars.

**Pararhizoclasia**

It is the inflammatory ulcerative destruction of the deep layers of tissue and the alveolar process around the root of a tooth.

**Parenteral**

Descriptive other methods of drug administration apart from the alimentary canal.

**Paresthesia**

The term refers to perverted sensation like burning, prickling or crawling sensation of the skin.

**Parodontal**

Near or next to a tooth sometimes used as synonymous with periodontal.

**Parrot tongue**

A horny, dry tongue which cannot be protruded. It is seen in typhus and low fever.

**Parulis**

It is mass of granulation tissue which covers the opening of a sinus.

**Pathogen**

Any agent that produces or is able to produce disease.

**Pathogenecity**

It is the ability of microbial species to produce disease.

**Pathogenesis**

The development of disease from its inception to the appearance of characteristic symptoms or lesions.

**Pathognomonic**

Characteristic of one specific disease or pathological condition as distinct from any others.

**Pathology**

That branch of medicine which is concerned with the structural and functional changes caused by disease.

**Pedunculated**

In this base of tumor is narrower than the most widest part of lesion.

**Percussion**

Listening to the tapping note with a finger placed on the affected part. In cases of teeth, it is done with the help of handle of the probe.

**Pericemental abscess**

A parodental abscess not arising from a diseased pulp or an extension of the periodontal pocket.

**Peridens**

Supernumerary teeth that are erupted ectopically either buccally or lingually to the normal arch referred to as peridens.

**Periodontal abscess**

An abscess that forms along the root of tooth perhaps following an advanced periodontal disease.

**Periodontitis**

It is name given to periodontal disease when the superficial inflammation in the gingival tissue extends into the underlying alveolar bone and there is loss of attachment.

**Periodontosis**

Chronic non-inflammatory destruction of periodontal ligament and its associated alveolar bone.

**Permeation**

The spreading or extension through tissues or organs, used especially of malignant tumors extending by continuous growth through the lymphatics.

**Petechiae**

Purpuric lesions 1–2 cm in diameter.

**Phlegmon**

Acute inflammation of the subcutaneous connective tissue.

**Phoenix abscess**

It is an acute exacerbation of a chronic or suppurative apical periodontitis.

**Pigmentation**

Pigmentation is a discoloration of the oral mucosa or gingiva due to the wide variety of lesions and conditions.

**Pilation**

It is a hair-like fracture found in cranial bones.

**Pit**

It is defined as hollow fovea or indent blind tracts lined with epithelium.

**Plasmapheresis**

It is a method of increasing the number of blood cells in the blood count from the blood plasma. They are skimmed out simply on standing and remaining concentrate is reinfused into the patient.

**Pleomorphic**

The word pleomorphic means occurring in several distinct shapes.

**Pleurodont**

Having teeth attached to the side of a bony socket or to the side of the jaw.

**Plexus**

A plexus of nerves or a network of blood or lymphatic vessels.

**Pocket**

It is an abnormal space developing between the tooth root and the gums.

**Poikiloderma**

It refers to a combination of atrophy, telangiectasia and pigmentary changes.

**Poison**

Any substance that when absorbed into the system of a living body is liable to cause injury and to endanger life.

**Polylophodont**

These are teeth with multi-ridged crowns.

**Pre-cancerous condition**

It is a generalized state associated with a significantly increased risk of cancer.

**Pre-cancerous lesion**

Morphologically altered tissue in which cancer is more likely to occur than its normal counterpart.

**Premedication**

The administration of drugs or sedatives before treatment, to help in patient management especially with nervous patient.

**Prescribe**

To write instruction for the preparation, composition and administration of a medicine.

**Prevalence**

The number of cases of a disease at any given time in any given place.

**Priestley's mass**

A green or brown stain on the anterior teeth of the young or where reduced enamel epithelium remains over the enamel.

**Procheilia**

It is the condition in which one lip protrudes forwards of its normal position.

**Prognosis**

It is the prediction of the course, duration and termination of the disease and the likelihood of its response to therapy.

**Prosthesis**

The word prosthesis is used for a manufactured appliance used to take the place of a natural part or to correct a congenital abnormality or it may be defined as an appliance which replaces lost or congenitally missing tissue.

**Proteolysis**

The process of digestion of proteins and its conversion by enzymes into peptones, proteoses, etc.

**Protuberance**

The word protuberance refers to a swelling, eminence or knob of the tissue.

**Pseudoepitheliomatous hyperplasia**

In this conditions the rete pegs extend far downward, usually accompanied by acanthosis. The cells are normal in size, shape and chromaticity.

**Pseudomembrane**

A false membrane, skin like layer formed by fibrinous exudates containing leukocytes and bacteria.

**Psychosomatic**

Relating to the mind and the body; particularly relating to the interdependence of mental processes and bodily function.

**Pulsation**

It is the rhythmic throb or beating as that of the heart.

**Pulse**

The expansion and contraction of an artery due to increased tension of its walls following contraction of the heart and subsequent relaxation.

**Purpura**

It refers to reddish to purple flat lesion caused by blood extravasated from a vessel leaking into subcutaneous tissue.

**Pus**

It is a liquid usually yellowish in color formed in certain infection and composed of tissue fluid containing bacteria and leukocytes.

**Pustule**

A raised lesion containing purulent material.

**Putrefaction**

The decomposition of organic matter through the action of microorganisms, resulting in the production of various solid and liquid compounds and gases giving off a foul odor.

**Pyemia**

Generalized septicemia caused by pyogenic microorganism in the bloodstream and marked by the formation of multiple abscesses.

**Radiology**

It is that branch of health sciences dealing with radioactive substances and radiant energy, with the diagnosis and treatment of diseases by means of both ionizing (X-rays) and non-ionizing (ultrasound) radiations.

**Radiolucent**

Offering little resistance to X-rays; appears almost transparent in radiography.

**Ranula**

The term ranula is used for a mucocele occurring in the floor of mouth in association with ducts of the submandibular or sublingual glands.

**Rash**

It refers to a temporary cutaneous eruption.

**Recrudescence**

The return of symptoms or the recurrence of the disease after a temporary remission.

**Recurrence**

The return of symptoms or of a disease after a period of remission.

**Regeneration**

It is replacement of injured tissue by parenchymal cells of the same types.

**Regurgitation**

The return of undigested or partially digested food from the stomach or oesophagus to the mouth or of fluid or semifluid to the nose.

**Reticular**

Relating to net or net-like structure.

**Retrogenia**

A condition in which chin is set back in relation to the rest of the facial skeleton.

**Rh hump**

In the deciduous 1$^{st}$ molar crown a characteristic ring-like defect may be seen which is called as Rh hump.

**Rhinorrhea**

Any discharge of fluid from the nose.

**Rhizotomy**

A surgical division of either a tooth root or a nerve root.

**Root dehiscence**

It is a pathological condition in which the vestibular surface of the tooth root is exposed to the oral cavity over some or all of the apical two-third of its length.

**Rubber jaw**

In this condition it is possible to mold the shape of the jaw with the fingers, but teeth will resume its position when the pressure is released.

**Rudiment**

It refers to an organ or part either imperfectly developed or at an early stage of development.

**Saburra**

It refers to a foul condition of the mouth and teeth or of the stomach due to food debris.

**Satellite abscess**

It is a secondary abscess arising from and situated near a primary abscess.

**Saucerization**

It is the wide and shallow depression occurring as a wound or bone cavity for example osteomyelitis.

**Scale**

Loosened, imperfectly cornified, parakeratotic superficial layer of skin that is shed as fine, brawny, dirty white and yellowish keratinous dust or large pearly white flakes.

**Sclerosis**

It refers to hardening of vessels or part applied particularly to arteries and proliferation of connective tissue in the nervous system as a result of degeneration.

**Septicemia**

The word septicemia implies a overwhelming bacterial proliferation and release of toxins in the blood.

**Sequestra**

Small pieces of necrotic bone which are avascular and which harbor microorganisms are known as sequestra.

**Serum**

If blood is allowed to clot an amber colored liquid which remains after separation of the clot is known as serum.

**Sessile**

Describing a tumor or growth whose base is the widest part of the lesion.

**Shock**

It is a state of inadequate perfusion of all cells and tissues, which at first leads to reversible hypoxic injury, but if insufficiently protracted or graved may lead to irreversible cell and organ injury and sometimes to the death of the patient.

**Sialolithiasis**

It is the formation of calcific concretions within parenchyma or ductal system of major or minor salivary glands.

**Sialorrhea (ptyalism)**

An increased salivary secretion is termed as sialorrhea or ptyalism.

**Sialoschesis**

It is the suppression of secretion of the salivary glands.

**Sickle cell anemia**

In homozygous individuals the whole of HbA (hemoglobin A) is replaced by HbS (hemoglobin S, i.e. an abnormal hemoglobin) and this is known as sickle cell disease.

**Sickle cell trait**

In heterozygous individuals, only 50% of HbA is replaced by HbS and this is known as sickle cell trait.

**Sign**

It is defined as any change in the body or its function which is perceptible to a trained observer and may indicate a specific disease.

**Sinus**

It is a blind tract leading from the surface down to the tissue which is lined by granulation tissue or which may be epithelized.

**Sinusitis**

Inflammation of mucosa of paranasal sinuses is referred to as sinusitis. When maxillary sinus is involved it is called as maxillary sinusitis.

**SLE (systemic lupus erythematous)**

It is characterised by the presence of abnormal serum antibodies and immune complexes.

**Slough**

It refers to the necrotizing tissue that scales or peels off in ulcerative conditions.

**Spongiosis**

This term is used to signify intercellular edema of the epithelium, in which intercellular bridges of the stratum spinosum are more prominent.

**Stagnation**

It refers to the cessation of flow of any circulating fluid in the body.

**Stenosis**

It is the constriction or narrowing of an aperture canal or duct.

**Sterile abscess**

An abscess containing no microorganisms.

**Sterilization**

It is the process of destruction of the microbial life from an article or surface inclusive of bacterial spores.

**Stimulus**

Any agent or impulse that excites or promotes a functional reaction.

**Stippled**

Having a mottled or spotted appearance with light and dark patches.

**Stomatology**

The medical speciality concerned with the mouth and its diseases sometimes used synonymously with dentistry.

**Striation**

It is a stripe or streak or a series of stripes or streaks.

**Stricture**

It is an abnormal contraction of any aperture or vessels.

**Stridor**

It is a harsh whistling sound produced by the respiratory system.

**Subluxation (hypermobility)**

It is the unilateral or bilateral positioning of the condyle anterior to the articular eminence, with repositioning to normal to accomplish normal physiologic activity.

**Subscription**

It is a part of a prescription containing direction for the preparation and compounding of the ingredients of a medicine.

**Superficially invasive (micro-invasive) squamous cell carcinoma**

A histopathological diagnosis of a routine squamous cell carcinoma, usually well differentiated, which has invaded only slightly into the underlying connective tissues.

**Suzanne's gland**

An oral mucous gland found in the alveololingual sulcus near the midline.

**Symbiosis**

It is the intimate association of two organism of different species.

**Symptoms**

Any indication of the presence or course of a disease either by functional or other changes occurring in the patient.

**Syncope**

It is a transient loss of consciousness caused by cerebral hypoxia or changes in cerebral blood flow.

**Syndesmosis**

It is the joining of two bone surfaces by the interposition of connective tissue which forms an interosseous membrane.

**Syndrome**

A complex of symptoms, occurring together, which characterize one disease or lesion.

**Tablet**

It is a small solid disc containing one dose of a drug.

**Talon's cusp**

It projects lingually from the cingulum area of maxillary and mandibular teeth. It is anomalous hyperplasia of cingulum on the lingual of maxillary and mandibular incisor resulting in the formation of a supernumerary cusp.

**Tapir mouth**

It is a condition characterised by loose thickened lips and caused by atrophy of the orbicularis oris muscle.

**Taste**

The perception of flavor, a sensation produced by stimulation of the gustatory nerve endings in the tongue with a soluble substance.

**Taurodontism**

Body of tooth is enlarged at the expense of root. It is characterised by clinical and anatomical crown of normal shape and size, an elongated body and short root with a longitudinally enlarged pulp chamber.

**Telangiectasia**

The dilatation of the capillaries and small arteries forming types of angiomas.

**Teratoma**

It is true neoplasm made up of a number of different types of tissue which are not native to the area in which the tumor occurs.

**Thalassemia**

It is an inherited impairment of hemoglobin synthesis in which there is partial or complete failure to synthesize a specific type of globin chain.

**Therapy**

It refers to the treatment of disease.

**Thermocautery**

It is the use of head points for cauterization.

**Tic**

A spasmodic twitching particularly of the facial muscles; a habit spasm.

**Tinnitus**

The term refers to a ringing noise in the ears.

**Toxin**

It is a poisonous substance produced by animal or vegetable cells more particularly by bacteria.

**Trabeculae**

It refers to a septum extending from the outer capsule or envelop into an organ.

**Transplantation**

It is the transfer of tissue either from another donor or from one site to another.

**Transposition**

It is the interchange in position of two adjacent teeth.

**Treatment**

It is the means used to combat or cure a disease.

**Trephone**

These are substances prepared by leukocytes from the plasma protein which is necessary for nourishment of tissue cell.

**Trignodent**

A tooth having three cusps in the form of a triangle.

**Trismus**

It is the inability to open the mouth because of tonic spasm of the jaw muscles.

**Trigeminal neuralgia (TN)**

It is defined as sudden, usually unilateral, severe, brief, stabbing, lancinating, paroxysmal, recurring pain in the distribution of one or more branches of 5th cranial nerve.

**Tropics**

It is that portion of the surface of the globe where the sun passes directly overhead.

**Tubercle**

It is a rounded eminence on bone.

**Tumefaction**

It is the state of being or becoming swollen.

**Tumor**

It is an autonomous new growth of tissue. It is an abnormal mass of tissue, the growth of which exceeds and is uncoordinated with that of normal tissue and persists in the same excessive manner even after the cessation of stimuli which evoked the change.

**Twining**

It indicates the cleavage of tooth germ into two complete tooth resulting in formation of supernumerary teeth that are mirror image or near image of tooth from which they have developed.

**Tyndallization**

A method of sterilizing culture media by exposure to steam at 100°C on three successive days for about 30 minutes each day.

**Ulcer**

Deep craters that extends through the entire thickness of the surface epithelium and involve the underlying connective tissue or defect in epithelium. It is a well circumscribed depressed lesion over which epidermal layer is lost.

**Unfavourable fracture**

If the associated muscle tends to pull the fragment of the fracture, it is described as unfavorable.

**Uvuloptosis**

It is a relaxed dropped position of palatine uvula.

**Vaccine**

It is any material used for preventive inoculation against a specific disease.

**Vallate**

Having a surrounding wall or rim.

**Varicosity**

A distended, superficial, bluish and painless vein.

**Vasodilator**

A nerve or some external agent which cause vascular dilatation.

**Verrucous**

In this tumor exhibits numerous surface projection.

**Vertigo**

It is a sensation of loss of equilibrium in which patients feel either that the world is revolving round them or that they are revolving in space.

**Vesicle**

These are elevated blisters containing clear fluid that are under 1 cm in diameter.

**Vicarious**

Relating to a normal process occurring in an abnormal position or under abnormal conditions.

**Virulence**

It is a term applied to the properties in a particular strain of microorganism.

**Virus**

A complex organic particle of submicroscopic dimensions capable of growth and reproduction only within the cells of the host organism it infects.

**Wandering abscess**

An abscess that tracks through the tissue and finally comes to a point some distance form the original site.

**Wandering teeth**

It is movement of unerupted teeth for no apparent reasons (distal drift).

**Wasting disease of teeth**

It is defined as any gradual loss of tooth substance characterised by the formation of smooth polished surfaces without ragged to the possible mechanism of this loss.

**Weal**

It is a reddish, raised and circumscribed lesion on the skin, generally caused by a blow or a bite.

**Wolff's law**

This law states that, the bone structure depends on the strain and stresses to which bone is subjected.

**Working diagnosis**

Following reappraisal of diagnostic data at hand, including those of follow-up examination which may be seen necessary and which may provide new relevant finding and indicating result from any additional diagnostic procedure.

**Wound**

It is any injury to the tissues or organs caused by cut, stab or tear, usually going deeper than the outer skin or integument.

**Xenograft**

It is a type of graft derived from a donor of different species.

**Xerostomia**

It is a subjective clinical condition of less than normal amount of saliva.

# Classifications

## Classifications of Vesiculobullous Lesions

Classification by Fitz and Patrick is as follows:

- According to anatomical plane
    - Intra epidermal blister granular layer
        - Pemphigus foliaceous
        - Frictional blisters
        - Staphylococcus scalded syndrome.
    - Spinous layer
        - Eczematous dermatitis
        - Secondary to heat and cold
        - Herpes virus infection
        - Familial benign pemphigus.
    - Suprabasal
        - Pemphigus vulgaris
        - Pemphigus vegetans
        - Darier's disease.
    - Basal layer
        - Erythema multiforme
        - Toxic epidermolysis necrolysis
        - Lupus erythematosis

  - Lichen planus
  - Epidermolysis bullosa simplex.

- Derma-epidermal junction zone
  - Lamina lucida
    - Bullous pemphigoid
    - Cicatricial pemphigoid
    - Epidermolysis bullosa junctional.
  - Below basal layer
    - Erythema multiforme
    - Epidermolysis bullosa dystrophica.

## Recurrent Aphthous Stomatitis

- Minor Aphthae
  - Also known as canker sores
  - Ulcers are less than 1 cm in diameter and they heal without a scar.
- Major Aphthae
  - It also known as periadenitis mucosa necrotica recurrent
  - Ulcers are 1 cm in diameter and heal with scarring.
- Herpetiform ulcers
  - Recurrent, many small ulcers are seen throughout the oral mucosa.
- Recurrent ulcers associates with behcet's syndrome

## Classification of White Lesions

- Variation in structure and appearance of the normal oral mucosa
  - Leukoedema
  - Fordyce's granules
  - Linea alba and other areas of frictional cornification.
- Non keratotic white lesion
  - Habitual cheek biting

- Burn (thermal, aspirin, dental medicaments, radiation mucositis & uraemic stomatitis)
- Caused by specific infectious agent (Koplik's spots, syphilitic patches).

❑ Candidiasis
- Acute pseudomembranous candidiasis (Oral Thrush)
- Acute atrophic candidiasis (Antibiotic sore mouth)
- Chronic Atrophic candidiasis (denture sore mouth and angular chelitis)
- Median rhomboid glossitis
- Chronic hyperplastic candidiasis.

❑ Keratotic white lesions with no increased potential for the development of oral cancer
- Stomatitis nicotina
- Traumatic keratosis
- Intra oral skin grafts
- Focal epithelial hyperplasia.
- Psoriasiform lesions (psoriasis, geographic tongue, Reiter syndrome).

❑ Red and White Lesion with defined or uncertain precancerous potential
- Leukoplakia (homogeneous, nodular or speckled and verrucous)
- Erythroplakia
- Oral Lesions with use of tobacco, betel nut chewing and snuff dipping tobacco (moist tobacco)
- Carcinoma in situ
- Oral submucous fibrosis
- Discoid lupus erythematosus
- Actinic keratosis
- Lichen planus
- Oral lichenoid Reactions.

## Classification of Oral Pigmentation

### ❑ Endogenous Pigmentations in Oral Mucosal Diseases

| Pigment | Colour | Disease |
|---|---|---|
| Hemoglobin | Blue/red/purple | Varix,hemangioma, kaposi's sarcoma,angiosarcoma |
| Hemosiderin | Brown | Ecchymosis, petechiae, thrombosed varix, hemorrhagic, mucocele,hemochromatosis |
| Melanin | Brown/black/ gray | Melanotic macule,nevus, melanoma, basilar melanosis with incontinence |

### ❑ Exogenous Pigmentations of Oral Mucosa

| Source | Colour | Disease |
|---|---|---|
| Silver amalgam | Gray/black | Tattoo, iatrogenic trauma |
| Graphite | Gray/black | Tattoo, trauma |
| Lead, Mercury, Bismuth | Gray | Ingestion of paint and medicines |

### ❑ Clinical Classification of Oral Pigmentation

| Colour | Solitary lesion | | Multiple lesion |
|---|---|---|---|
| | Focal lesion | Diffuse lesion | |
| Blue/ purple | Varix, hemangioma | Hemangioma | Kaposi's sarcoma,hereditary hemorrhagic telangiectasia |
| Brown | Melanotic macule, nevus, melanoma | Ecchymosis, melanoma, hairy tongue, drug induced | Physiologic pigment, neurofibromatosis, hemochromatosis, Addison's disease, drug induced, Peutz-jeghers syndrome, petechiae |

*Contd.*

*Contd.*

| Colour | Solitary lesion | | Multiple lesion |
|---|---|---|---|
| | **Focal lesion** | **Diffuse lesion** | |
| Gray/ black | Amalgam, nevus, graphite, melanoma | Amalgam, melanoma, hairy tongue | Heavy metal ingestion |

## Classification of Osteosarcoma

- ❑ Chondroblastic
- ❑ Osteoblastic
- ❑ Fibroblastic

## WHO Classification for Precancerous Lesions and Conditions

| Precancerous lesions | Precancerous conditions |
|---|---|
| Leukoplakia | Submucous fibrosis |
| Erythroplakia | Actinic keratosis |
| Palatal lesions in reverse smokers | Lichen planus , Discoid lupus erythematosus |

## Classification of Salivary Gland Tumors

- ❑ Benign
  - Mixed tumor
  - Papillary cystadenoma lymphomatosum
  - Oxyphilic adenoma
  - Sebaceous cell adenoma
  - Benign lymphoepithelial lesion
  - Unclassified.
- ❑ Malignant
  - Malignant mixed tumor
  - Mucoepidermoid tumor; low grade and high grade
  - Squamous cell carcinoma

- Adenocarcinoma
- Adenoid cystic carcinoma
- Trabecular or solid
- Anaplastic
- Mucous cell
- Pseudoadamantine adenocarcinoma
- Acinic cell carcinoma
- Unclassified.

❑ Revised Classification WHO 1991

- Adenomas
  - Pleomorphic adenoma
  - Myoepithelioma (myoepithelial adenoma)
  - Warthin's tumour (Adenolymphoma)
  - Oncocytoma (oncocytic adenoma)
  - Basal cell adenoma
  - Canalicular adenoma
  - Sebaceous adenoma
  - Ductal papilloma
    - Inverted ductal papilloma
    - Intraductal papilloma
    - Sialadenoma papilliferum.
- Cystadenoma
  - Papillary cyst adenoma
  - Mucinous cyst adenoma
- Carcinomas
  - Acinic cell carcinoma
  - Mucoepidermoid carcinoma
  - Adenoid cystic carcinoma
  - Epithelial – myoepithelial carcinoma
  - Polymorphous low grade adenocarcinom
  - Basal cell adenocarcinoma
  - Mucinous adenocarcinoma
  - Papillary cyst adenocarcinoma
  - Oncocytic carcinoma
  - Salivary duct carcinoma

- Adenocarcinoma
- Malignant myoepithelioma
- Carcinoma in pleomorphic adenoma (malignant mixed tumour)
- Squamous cell carcinoma
- Small cell carcinoma
- Undifferentiated carcinoma.

- Other carcinomas
- Non epithelial tumours
- Malignant lymphomas
- Secondary tumours
- Unclassified tumours
- Tumour like lesions
  - Sialadenosis
  - Oncocytosis
  - Nectrotizing sialometaplasia (salivary gland infarction)
  - Benign lymphoepithelial lesion
  - Salivary gland cysts
  - Chronic sclerosing sialadenitis of submandibular gland (kuttner tumour)
  - Cystic lymphoid hyperplasia in AIDS.

## Classification of Temporomandibular Joint Disorders

- Extrinsic extra-articular disorders
  - Masticatory muscle disorders
    - Protective muscle splinting
    - Masticatory muscle spasm
    - Masticatory muscle inflammation.
  - Extrinsic trauma
    - Traumatic arthritis
    - Tendonitis
    - Fracture
    - Myositis
    - Internal disc derangement
    - Contracture of elevator muscle.

- Intrinsic/intra-articular disorders
  - Trauma
    - Dislocation, subluxation
    - Haemarthrosis
    - Intracapsular f racture, extracapsular fracture.
  - Internal disc displacement
    - Anterior disc displacement with reduction.
    - Anterior disc displacement without reduction.
  - Arthritis
    - Osteoarthritis.
    - Rheumatoid arthiritis.
    - Juvenile rheumatoid arthritis
    - Infectious arthritis.
  - Developmental defects
    - Condylar agenesis or aplasia-unilateral or bilateral
    - Condylar hypoplasia
    - Condylar hyperplasia.
  - Ankylosis
  - Neoplasms
    - Benigh tumours: osteoma, osteochondroma, chondroma
    - Malignant tumours: chondrosarcoma, fibrosarcoma, synovial sarcoma.

## Classification of Dislocation/Subluxation

- Acute
- Chronic
- Long standing.

## Classification of Ankylosis

- False ankylosis or true ankylosis
- Extra-articular or intra-articular
- Fibrous or bony
- Unilateral or bilateral
- Partial or complete.

## Grading of Tmj Ankylosis

- Sawhney Grading of TMJ Ankylosis
  - Type I: Condylar head is normal without much distortion, Fibrous adhesions make movement impossible.
  - Type II: Bony fusion of the distorted condylar head and the articular surface. No involvement of sigmoid notch and coronoid process
  - Type III: Bony bridging block from lateral ramus to zygomatic arch. Medially an atrophic dislocated fragment of the former head of the condyle is still found. Elongation of the coronoid process is seen.
  - Type IV: Normal anatomy of TMJ is completely destroyed by complete bony block between ramus and skull base.

## Classification of Regressive Alteration of Teeth

- Tooth wear
  - Attrition
  - Abrasion
  - Erosion (corrosion)
  - Abfraction.
- Teeth resorption
  - External
  - Internal.
- Dentinal changes
  - Reparative dentinal
  - Secondary dentinal
  - Dead tracts.
- Cemental Changes
  - Cementicles
  - Hypercementosis.
- Pulpal Changes
  - Reticular Atropy of Pulp
  - Pulp Clasification.

## Classification of Odontogenic and Non Odontogenic Tumors

- Benign odontogenic tumours of the jaws (Kramer, Pindborg, Shear classification):
  - Odontogenic epithelium without odontogenic ectomesenchyme
    - Ameloblastoma
    - Calicifying epithelial odontogenic tumour–CEOT, Pindborg's tumour
    - Clear cell odontogenic tumour
    - Squamous odontogenic tumour.
  - Odontogenic epithelium with odontogenic ectomesenchyme with or without dental hard tissue formation
    - Ameloblastic fibroma
    - Ameloblastic fibrodentinoma
    - Odontoameloblastoma
    - Adenomatoid odontogenic tumour (AOT)
    - Complex Odontome
    - Compound odontome.
  - Odontogenic ectomesenchyme with or without odontogenic epithelium
    - Odontogenic fibroma
    - Myxoma (odontogenic myxoma, myxofibroma)
    - Benign cementoblastoma (true cementoma).
- Classification of odontogenic tumours (Gorlin, Chaudhary, Pindborg)
  - Epithelial odontogenic tumours
    - Minimal inductive change in connective tissue (Ectodermal origin)
      - Ameloblastoma
      - Adenomatoid odontogenic tumour
      - Calcifying epithelial odontogenic tumour (CEOT).

- Marked inductive change in connective tissue (Mixed agents)
  - Ameloblastic fibroma
  - Ameloblastic odontoma
  - Odontoma
  - Complex odontoma
  - Compound odontoma.
- Mesodermal odontogenic tumours
  - Odontogenic myxoma
  - Odontogenic fibroma
  - Cementoma
    - Periapical cemental dysplasia
    - Benign cementoblastoma
    - Cementifying fibroma
    - Familial multiple (gigantiform) cementoma
    - Florid osseous dysplasia-FOD.

❑ Non-odontogenic tumours and fibro-osseous lesions of the jaw bones

- Non- odontogenic tumours
  - Central fibroma
  - Myxofibroma
  - Ossifying fibroma
  - Osteoma
  - Osteoid osteoma
  - Benign osteoclastoma
  - Chondroma
  - Giant cell granuloma
  - Central hemangioma
  - Benign tumours of nerve tissue.
- Fibro-osseous lesions
  - Fibrous dysplasia of bone
  - Cherubism (Inherited fibro osseous bone disease)
  - Ossifying fibroma
  - Central giant cell granuloma.

## Classification of Non-Odontogenic Tumours of the Jaws (Kramer, Pindborg, Shear)

- Osteogenic neoplasms
  - Cemento-ossifying fibroma.
- Non-neoplastic bone lesions
  - Fibrous dysplasia of the jaws
  - Cemento- osseous dysplasia
    - Periapical cemento osseous dysplasia
    - Focal cemento osseous dysplasia
    - Florid cemento osseous dysplasia (gigantiform).
- Other cemento- osseous dysplasias
  - Cherubism
  - Central giant cell granuloma.

## Classification of Nerve Injuries

Seddon's Classification

- Grade 1-mildest or neurapraxia
- Grade 2-severe or axonotmesis
- Grade 3-most severe or neurotmesis.

## Classification of Oral Candidiasis

- Pseudomembranous candidiasis/oral thrush
- Erythematous candidiasis
- Hyperplastic candidiasis
- Angular cheilitis.

## Classification of Diabetes

- Type I–it is also known as Insulin dependent diabetes
- Type II–it is also known as Non insulin dependent diabetes.

## Classification of Anemia

Etiological Classification of Anemia

- Loss of Blood

- Acute post hemorrhagic anemia
- Chronic post hemorrhagic anemia.

❑ Excessive destruction of RBCs
- Extracorpuscular causes
  - Antibodies
  - Infections like malaria
  - Splenic sequestration and destruction
  - Associated diseases like lymphomas
  - Drugs, chemical and physical agents
  - Trauma to RBC.
- Intracorpuscular hemolytic diseases
  - Hereditary :
    - Disorders of glycolysis
    - Erythropoietic purpura
    - Faulty synthesis or maintenance of reduced glutoathione
    - Qualitative or quantitative abnormalities in the synthesis of globulin
    - Abnormalities in RBC membrane.
  - Acquired:
    - Paroxysmal nocturnal hemoglobinuria
    - Lead poisoning.

❑ Impaired blood production resulting from deficiency of substances essential for erythropoiesis
- Iron deficiency
- Deficiency of Vit. B12, ↓ folic acid
- Pyridoxine responsive anemia
- Protein deficiency
- Ascorbic acid deficiency.

❑ Inadequate production of immature erythrocytes
- Deficiency of erythroblast
  - Aplastic anemia
    - Chemical or physical agents
    - Hereditary
    - Idiopathic.

    - Pure red cell aplasia
        - Thymoma
        - Chemical agents
        - Antibodies.
- Infiltration of bone marrow
    - Leukemia
    - Multiple myeloma
    - Carcinoma
    - Sarcoma
    - Myelofibrosis.
- Endocrine abnormalities
    - Myxedema
    - Addison's diseases
    - Pituitary insufficiency
    - Hyperthyroidism.
- Chronic renal failure
- Chronic inflammatory dieases
    - Infectious
    - Non infectious.
- Cirrhosis of liver.

Morphologic Classification

- ❑ Macrocytic Anemia: Increased MCV, MCH and normal MCH conc
- ❑ Normocytic Anemia: reduction in RBC membrane, normal MCV, MCH and MCH conc
- ❑ Simple microcytic: reduced MCV, MCH and MCH conc
- ❑ Hypochromic microcytic: reduced MCV, MCH and MCH conc.

## Classification of Leukemia

- ❑ Acute
    - Acute lymphoblastic leukemia
        - L1: Acute lymphoblastic (principally pediatric)-small cells predominate and nuclei are round

- L2: Acute lymphoblastic (principally adults)–cells are heterogenous in size and sharp in features, nuclei often show cleft
- L3: Homogenous population of large cells. Nuclei are round to oval and have prominent nucleoli.

- Acute non-lymphoblastic or myeloid leukemia
  - M1-Myeloblastic (without maturation)–myeloblasts predominate with distant nucleoli, few granules are present
  - M2-myeloblastic ( with maturation)-myeloblasts and promyelocytes predominate and Auer rods can be seen
  - M3-Promyelocytic- hypergranular promyelocytes often with Auer rods are seen
  - M4-Myelomonocytic-myelocytic and monocytic differentiation is evident, myeloid elements resemble peripheral monocytosis
  - M5-Monocytic–promonocytes or undifferentiated blasts
  - M6-Erythroleukemia–bizzare, multinucleated, megablastoid erythroblast predominate
  - M7-Megakaryocytic-pleomorphic undifferentiated blast cells with anti-platelet antibodies, myelofibrosis is seen.

❑ Chronic
- Chronic lymphocytic leukemia
- Chronic myeloid leukemia.

## Classify Tongue Diseases

❑ Congenital and developmental disorders
- Aglossia and microglossia
- Macroglossia
- Ankyloglossia

- Cleft tongue
- Ankyloglossum superius syndrome
- Lingual varices
- Lingual thyroid nodule
- Variations in tongue movement
- Thyroglossal duct cyst
- Tongue thrusting
- Lingual polyp
- Reactive lymphoid aggregates
- Lingual cyst.

❑ Local tongue disorders
- Median rhomboid glossitis
- Fissured tongue
- Benign migratory glossitis
- Hairy tongue
- Foliate papillitis.

❑ Depapillation of tongue
- Local disease
    - Eosinophilic granuloma
    - Traumatic injuries
    - Lesions due to auto mutilations
    - Allergic stomatitis
    - Facial hemiatrophy
    - Cranial arteritis
    - Chronic candidiasis.
- Systemic disease
    - Iron deficiency anemia
    - Plummer Vinson syndrome
    - Pernicious anemia
    - Niacin deficiency
    - Folic acid deficiency
    - Peripheral vascular disease
    - Dermatomyositis
    - Diabetes

  - Syphilis
  - Zoster infection
  - Tuberculosis.
- ❑ Neurological disease
  - Glossodynia
  - Paralysis
  - Dyskinesia
  - Oropharyngeal dysphagia.
- ❑ Cyst
  - Bronchogenic cyst
  - Anterior median lingual cyst
  - Gastric mucosal cyst
  - Epidermoid and dermoid cyst
  - Thyroglossal cyst
  - Parasitic cyst.
- ❑ Benign tumor
  - Fibroma
  - Granular cell tumor
  - Glomus tumor
  - Leiomyoma
  - Plasmacytoma
  - Rhabdomyoma.
- ❑ Premalignant lesion and condition
  - Leukoplakia
  - Lichen planus
  - Oral Submucous Fibrosis (OSMF).
- ❑ Malignant tumor
  - Squamous cell carcinoma
  - Malignant lymphoma
  - Malignant melanoma
  - Metastatic tumor
  - Sarcoma.
- ❑ Miscellaneous
  - Phlebectasia
  - Pigmentation of tongue.

# Viva-Voce

1. **Which transplant patient is more prone to have dental caries?**

**Ans:** Hematopoietic cell transplantation

2. **Which drugs are associated with drug-induced gingival overgrowth?**

**Ans:** Cyclosporine, Nifedipine and Phenytoin

3. **Multiresistant herpes simplex virus infection can be successfully treated by**

**Ans:** Foscarnet

4. **Which oro-dental manifestations may be present in children who have undergone hematopoietic cell transplantation?**

**Ans:** Dental caries, altered root formation and dentofacial abnormalities

5. **The best time to perform elective dental treatment in post-transplantation patient is**

**Ans:** Stable period

6. **Which neoplasm is more likely to develop in transplant recipients?**

**Ans:** Kaposi's sarcoma

7. **"Wispy hyperkeratosis on an erythematous base" on the oral mucosa of the patient who has undergone hematopoietic cell transplantation is due to?**

**Ans:** Graft-versus-host disease

8. **Graft-versus-host disease in the oral mucous membrane can be treated by**

**Ans:** Topical cyclosporine and topical azathioprine

9. **The most common viral pathogen cultured from oral infection in transplant recipient is**

**Ans:** Herpes simplex virus

10. **"Brittle insulin-dependent diabetes" may be found in patients awaiting**

**Ans:** Pancreatic transplantation

11. **Virus that causes oral ulcerations in immunosuppressed patient is**

**Ans:** Herpes simplex virus

12. **History of prodromal symptoms preceding the local lesions is found in**

**Ans:** Herpes virus infection

13. **Acyclovir controls herpes simplex infections by**

**Ans:** Inhibiting DNA replication in HSV infected cells

14. **Acute lymphonodular pharyngitis is caused by**

**Ans:** Coxsackie A10

**15. The required adult oral dose of acyclovir in the treatment of severe herpes zoster is**

**Ans:** 800 mg five times daily

**16. Large, irregular, deep and bleeding ulcers in the oral cavity are found in**

**Ans:** Erythema multiforme

**17. Necrotic, punched out ulcerations are the clinical features of**

**Ans:** ANUG

**18. Hyper-reactivity to intracutaneous injection or a needlestick is found in the patients of**

**Ans:** Behcet's disease

**19. Nikolsky's sign is most frequently associated with**

**Ans:** Pemphigus

**20. Use of corticosteroid is contraindicated in**

**Ans:** Primary herpes

**21. Formation of symblepharon and corneal damage is common in**

**Ans:** Mucous membrane pemphigoid

**22. Indolent lesions of erosive lichen planus can be treated by**

**Ans:** Intralesional steroids

**23. Name one non-keratotic lesion?**

**Ans:** Uremic stomatitis

**24. What is not a histological feature of leukoedema?**

**Ans:** Keratinization

**25. The number of Fordyces granules present on oral mucosa**

**Ans:** Increases with age

**26. Uremic stomatitis is caused in seriously ill patients with renal failure and blood urea nitrogen level**

**Ans:** More than 250 mg/d

**27. Denture sore-mouth is**

**Ans:** Rarely found under the mandibular denture

**28. Dental hypoplasia and severe caries are common in**

**Ans:** Candidiasis endocrinopathy syndrome

**29. Which lesion does not have precancerous potential?**

**Ans:** Keratosis follicularis

**30. "Monro's abscesses" are found in**

**Ans:** Psoriasis

**31. Orifices of palatal minor salivary glands appear as white, umblicated nodules with red centers in**

**Ans:** Stomatitis nicotina palati

**32. White epithelial pearls' or 'tobacco cells" or "cells-within-cells" occur most extensively in the cytologic examination of**

**Ans:** Hereditary benign intra-epithelial dyskeratosis

**33. "Grains and "corps ronds" can be examined in the cytologic smear of**

**Ans:** Keratosis follicularis

**34. Mixed red and white lesions are found in**

**Ans:** Nodular leukoplakia

**35. Major causative factor of leukoplakia is**

**Ans:** Tobacco

**36. Which site in the mouth has highest rate for malignant transformation of oral leukoplakia?**

**Ans:** Floor of mouth

**37. Which diseases are correlated with tobacco use?**

**Ans:** Frictional keratosis, leukoedema and hairy tongue

**38. White patches surrounded by a telangiectatic halo are found in**

**Ans:** Discoid lupus erythematosus

**39. "Wickham's striae" are found in**

**Ans:** Reticular from of lichen planus

**40. An association between oral lichen planus, diabetes mellitus and hypertension is found in which syndrome?**

**Ans:** Grinspan's syndrome

**41. Which disease does not exhibit Lichenoid tissue reaction?**

**Ans:** Leukoplakia

**42. Which syndrome is associated with vascular lesions?**

**Ans:** Sturge-Weber syndrome

**43. Name a non brown melanotic lesion?**

**Ans:** Varices

**44. The most common oral site for Kaposi's sarcoma is**

**Ans:** Palate

**45. Which is multifocal pigmentation of oral tissue?**

**Ans:** Hemochromatosis

**46. In the oral mucosa ,which colour does blue nevi tend to exhibit?**

**Ans:** Blue colour

**47. Which drug produces oral pigmentation?**

**Ans:** Minocycline

**48. "Café au lait" pigmentations are found in**

**Ans:** Neurofibromatosis

**49. What causes patchy melanosis of the oral mucosa in Addison's disease?**

**Ans:** Increased secretion of ACTH

**50. The most frequently affected site of HIV oral melanosis is**

**Ans:** Buccal mucosa

**51. Which is the most common source of focal pigmentation in the oral mucosa?**

**Ans:** Amalgam tattoo

**52. Name the site where pigmentation due to heavy mental ingestion is usually found?**

**Ans:** Along the free gingival margin

**53. Typical oral Kaposi's sarcoma lesions are**

**Ans:** Multifocal

**54. Structural variants clinically appearing as slightly red nodular elevations are known as**

**Ans:** Oral tonsils

**55. The inflammatory hyperplasia will not recur if**

**Ans:** Irritant is eliminated with excision of lesion

**56. Lesions developing on the hard palate due to dentures with relief areas or "suction chambers" are known as**

**Ans:** Palatal papillomatosis

**57. Pyogenic granuloma gradually converts into fibrous epulis when it becomes?**

**Ans:** Less vascular and more collagenous

**58. Name one lesion that is not a benign fibro-osseous lesion?**

**Ans:** Osteitis deformans

**59. Cysts containing hair follicles, sweat glands and sebum are called as**

**Ans:** Epidermoid cyst

**60. Name a tumor of mesodermal origin?**

**Ans:** Cementifying fibroma

**61. Tumor occurring usually in children under six months of age is**

**Ans:** Melanoameloblastoma

**62. Virus-induced tumor characterized by soft, sessile papules is found in**

**Ans:** Heck's disease

**63. "Floating teeth" are found in**

**Ans:** Langerhan's cell granulomatosis

**64. The most frequent site of involvement in cervicofacial actinomycosis is**

**Ans:** Submandibular region

**65. Mouth breathers mainly exhibit gingival enlargements in**

**Ans:** Maxillary anterior region

**66. Cyst that remains attached to the neck of the tooth enclosing the crown within the cyst is**

**Ans:** Dentigerous cyst

**67. The size of cervical lymph node of stage N2B is**

**Ans:** Less than 6 cm

**68. Virus most commonly present in oral squamous cell carcinoma is**

**Ans:** HPV type 16

**69. Treatment of choice for exophytic and well-oxygenated tumor is**

**Ans:** Radiotherapy

**70. Primary tumor of posterior third of the tongue is best treated by**

**Ans:** External beam therapy

**71. Total dose of radiations given for treatment of malignant tumor is**

**Ans:** 6000–6500 cGY

**72. The most common symptom of nasopharyngeal carcinoma is**

**Ans:** Neck mass

**73. Most rapidly increasing malignant disease in AIDS is**

**Ans:** Lymphoma

**74. Which drug can be used prophylactically to reduce complications of radiotherapy?**

**Ans:** Benzydamine HCI

**75. What is not a complication of radiation therapy?**

**Ans:** Parotitis

**76. Bowen's disease occurs on skin as a result of**

**Ans:** Arsenic ingestion

**77. Which syndrome has findings of cleft lip, cleft palate and congenital lip pit?**

**Ans:** Van der Woude's syndrome

**78. Tongue with thick leathery coating in dehydrated and debilitated patients is referred to as**

**Ans:** Earthy tongue

**79. Non-ulcerating, irregular indurations on the tongue with leukoplakia are seen in**

**Ans:** Interstitial glossitis

**80. Series of ulcers along the anterior third of the tongue on one side are seen in**

**Ans:** Herpes zoster infection

**81. Purplish blue spots, nodules and ridges on anterior ventral surface of the tongue are referred to as**

**Ans:** Lingual varicosities

**82. Lipoprotein lipase needed for digestion of fat in infants is secreted from**

**Ans:** Glands of von Ebner

**83. Rapid repetitive uncontrolled movement of the tongue is called as**

**Ans:** Tardive dyskinesia

**84. Majority of tongue carcinomas occur on**

**Ans:** Anterior two-third of the tongue

**85. Carcinoma of the posterior tongue is mostly treated by**

**Ans:** Radiation

**86. "Long and narrow" tongue as a result of hyperostosis and thickening of the mandible is seen in**

**Ans:** Tuberous sclerosis

**87. Riga's ulcers on the tongue of the infants occur on**

**Ans:** Lingual frenum

**88. "Strawberry tongue" is a classic sign, found in infection with**

**Ans:** Streptococcus pyogenes

**89. Annular circinate and serpiginous lesions of the tongue are found in**

**Ans:** Geographic tongue

**90. Where is an aberrant salivary gland found?**

**Ans:** Posterior to the first molar near the body of mandible

**91. Sialoliths most frequently occur in**

**Ans:** Sub-mandibular gland

**92. Mucous-extravasation cysts are usually found on**

**Ans:** Lower lip

**93. In sialadenitis, viscosity and turbidity of the saliva**

**Ans:** Increases

**94. Name a non-inflammatory disease of salivary gland?**

**Ans:** Sialadenosis

**95. Acute non-suppurative parotitis can be caused by**

**Ans:** Paramyxovirus, parainfluenza type 1 and parainfluenza type 3

**96. Purulent discharge with sulphur granules is milked from salivary gland duct when it is infected by**

**Ans:** Actinomycosis

**97. Chemical constituents of salivary flow are characterized by**

**Ans:** Increased salivary K and decreased salivary Na

**98. A "salt and pepper" appearance of the salivary glands on MRI suggests**

**Ans:** Sjogren's syndrome

**99. Disorder associated with decreased salivary flow in debilitated patient is**

**Ans:** Acute parotitis

**100. Dose of intraductal erythromycin for the treatment of chronic nonspecific bacterial sialadenitis is**

**Ans:** 15 mg/ml for 5 days

**101. The lateral mandibular motion ranges from**

**Ans:** 8–10 mm

**102. The muscles most often involved in MPDS are**

**Ans:** Temporalis and geniohyoid

**103. Ely's cyst is found in**

**Ans:** Septic arthritis

**104. Chronic pain or pain of increased intensity due to internal derangements in the TMJ can be treated by**

**Ans:** Mandibular protrusive splint

**105. Synovial chondromatosis is characterized by**

**Ans:** Cartilaginous nodules of the synovial membrane

**106. Micrognathia and anterior open bite are found in**

**Ans:** Juvenile rheumatoid arthritis

**107. Pitting of the nails is a characteristic clinical feature of**

**Ans:** Psoriatic arthritis

**108. Large and tender cervical lymph nodes are found in**

**Ans:** Septic arthritis

**109. Flatness of face on one side is found in**

**Ans:** Condylar hypoplasia

**110. Unilateral pain in perauricular region, which becomes worse on awakening is a clinical features of?**

**Ans:** Myofascial pain dysfunction syndrome

**111. Painful syndrome characterized by faulty identification and localization of stimulus is**

**Ans:** Hyperpathia

**112. The recommended dose of carbamazepine for treatment of trigeminal neuralgia is**

**Ans:** Initial dose of 200 mg/day increased to 800–1200 mg/day

**113. Geniculate neuralgia results from herpetic inflammation of**

**Ans:** Cranial nerve VII

**114. Conjunctival reddening is observed in**

**Ans:** Cluster headache

**115. Drug used prophylactically for preventing migraine headache is**

**Ans:** Propranolol

**116. "Claudication" of the masticatory muscles is found in**

**Ans:** Cranial arteritis

**117. Cluster headache is triggered by**

**Ans:** Smoking

**118 Signs and symptoms present is stage 2 sympathetic dystrophy are**

**Ans:** Cold intolerance, hyperesthetic pain and decreased skin temperature

**119. Loss of the ability to classify or identify a given taste stimulus refers to**

**Ans:** Gustatory agnosia

**120. What is not a "true taste disorder"?**

**Ans:** Secondary dysgeusias

**121. Familial dysautonomia is a rare disorder associated with**

**Ans:** Hypersalivation, abnormal taste sensation and excessive sweating

**122. Deficiency of which mineral is associated with taste dysfunction?**

**Ans:** Zinc

**123. Olfactory and gustatory sensations are lost in head injury due to damage to**

**Ans:** Temporal lobe

**124. Risk of coronary heart disease can be reduced by**

**Ans:** Raising LDL level and lowering HDL level

**125. Chest pain occurring at rest mostly at night or during ordinary activity is**

**Ans:** Variant angina

**126. Severe crushing pain in the left side of the jaw that is brought on by exertion and is relieved by rest and lasts for few seconds to few minutes is seen in**

**Ans:** Angina pectoris

**127. The skin eruptions found in rheumatic fever are known as**

**Ans:** Erythema marginatum

**128. Characteristic clinical feature found in endocarditis is**

**Ans:** Petechial haemorrhage in the conjunctivae

**129. Cardiac condition in which endocarditis prophylaxis is not recommended before dental treatment is?**

**Ans:** Cardiac pacemakers

**130. Drug of choice for patient with rheumatic heart disease undergoing surgical procedure in the oral cavity is**

**Ans:** Amoxicillin

**131. Diastolic pressure in stage-2 hypertension ranges between**

**Ans:** 100–109 mm Hg

**132. Antihypertensive drug that may cause gingival enlargement is**

**Ans:** Diltiazem

**133. Cyanosis of the oral mucosa with severe marginal gingivitis is clinical feature in**

**Ans:** Tetralogy of Fallot

**134. The early sings of congestive heart failure are**

**Ans:** Cyanosis of the oral mucosa with ankle edema

**135. Which antihypertensive drug may cause ulcerations in the oral mucous membrane?**

**Ans:** Methyldopa

**136. Microorganisms responsible for sinusitis particularly in children**

**Ans:** Streptococcus pneumoniae, streptococcus aureus and streptococcus pyogenes

**137. Long duration hoarseness of voice with acute pain and dysphagia is found in**

**Ans:** Tuberculous laryngitis

**138. The commonest cause of chronic bronchitis is**

**Ans:** Smoking

**139. In immunosuppressed patients, pneumonia is mostly caused by**

**Ans:** Pneumocystis carinii

**140. Drug of choice for treatment of pneumocystis carinii pneumonia is**

**Ans:** Pentamidine

**141. Which infectious disease is also referred to as "acid-fast infection"?**

**Ans:** Tuberculosis

**142. Scrofula refers to**

**Ans:** Tuberculous involvement of cervical lymph nodes

**143. Oral lesions in tuberculosis are characterized by**

**Ans:** Small ulcers at the corners of the mouth, lesions at the lateral margin of the tongue and deep central ulcers of the tongue

**144. Dental treatment in actively infected patient with tuberculosis can be carried out**

**Ans:** After 3 months of antitubercular therapy

**145. The most presenting oral manifestation of Wegener's granulomatosis is**

**Ans:** Hemorrhagic gingival enlargement

**146. Destruction and perforation of hard and soft palates are found in**

**Ans:** Midline granuloma

**147. Tetracycline staining of the teeth is commonly seen in patients of**

**Ans:** Cystic fibrosis

**148. Swallowing tablets or capsules without adequate amount of water may lead to**

**Ans:** Esophageal ulcer

**149. What is the most frequent cause of peptic ulceration?**

**Ans:** Infection with Helicobacter pylori

**150. Which drug used in the treatment of peptic ulcer may lead to xerostomia?**

**Ans:** Atropine

**151. Which drug used may induce hepatitis?**

**Ans:** Isoniazid hydrochloride

**152. Yellow discoloration of oral mucosa in hepatitis is most readily seen on**

**Ans:** Palate

**153. Chronic hepatitis B can be treated by administration of**

**Ans:** Interferon alpha-2b

**154. Oral manifestation in Crohn's disease is characterized by**

**Ans:** Aphthous like ulcerations

**155. Hepatic dysfunction or severe jaundice may lead to**

**Ans:** Severe bleeding following periodontal operation and spontaneous bleeding in the oral cavity

**156. Which method is not effective in inactivating hepatitis B virus?**

**Ans:** Immersion in solution of isopropyl alcohol for 15 minutes

**157. Least amount of infected blood on dental instruments that may transmit hepatitis virus to dental surgeon and other patients is**

**Ans:** 0.0004 ml

**158. Which is the second most common cause of renal failure?**

**Ans:** Pyelonephritis

**159. Changes associated with renal osteodystrophy are most frequently seen in**

**Ans:** Mandibular molar region

**160. The giant cell lesions found in hyperparathyroidism and related to renal diseases are called as**

**Ans:** Brown tumor

**161. Which is not an oral manifestation in dialysis patients?**

**Ans:** Enamel hypoplasia

**162. Uremic stomatitis occurs in oral cavity when**

**Ans:** Bun level is greater than 150 mg/dl

**163. Dental treatment of patient with renal disease should be performed**

**Ans:** Within 24 hours of dialysis

**164. The recommended dose of prednisone used for antirejection therapy in kidney transplantation is**

**Ans:** 10–40 mg/day

**165. Administration of cyclosporine in kidney transplant patients may lead to**

**Ans:** Hepatic dysfunction, kidney arteriolopathy and gingival hyperplasia

**166. Which drug can produce stomatitis and xerostomia?**

**Ans:** Azathioprine

**167. The first and most frequently involved area of cyclosporine-induced gingival hyperplasia is**

**Ans:** Labial gingiva in the anterior teeth

**168. X-linked agammaglobulinemia is caused by defect in**

**Ans:** B-cell function

**169. B-lymphocyte deficiencies are associated with**

**Ans:** Bacterial infections

**170. Congenital defects of the mouth and jaws are seen in**

**Ans:** X-linked agammaglobulinemia, severe combined immunodeficiency and secondary immune deficiency

**171. AIDS patients become susceptible to infections when T4 lymphocytes count is below**

**Ans:** 50 mm3

**172. Persistent generalized lymphadenopathy occurs in AIDS patients during**

**Ans:** Asymptomatic phase

**173. An initial opportunistic infection in AIDS patients is of**

**Ans:** Pneumocystis carinii pneumonia

**174. The second most common tumor in AIDS patients is**

**Ans:** Non-Hodgkin's lymphoma

**175. The drug used in management of AIDS is**

**Ans:** Azidothymidine, pentamidine and didanosine

**176. Hard and rigid tongue and lips with narrow mouth opening are oral finding in**

**Ans:** Rheumatoid arthritis

**177. Which muscles get weakened in dermatomyositis?**

**Ans:** Palatal muscles

**178. The recommended dose of epinephrine for treatment of generalized anaphylaxis in adults is**

**Ans:** 0.5 ml intravenously

**179. Uniform thickening of periodontal ligament around posterior teeth is found in**

**Ans:** Linear localized scleroderma

**180. The most frequent site of brain involvement in cerebral abscess due to odontogenic infection is**

**Ans:** Frontal lobe

**181. Impairment of vision, muscular incoordination and bladder dysfunction are found in**

**Ans:** Multiple sclerosis

**182. Rapid vision loss following an increase in body temperature associated with heavy exercise is known as**

**Ans:** Uhthoff's sign

**183. Impaired swallowing or paresthesia of the mouth and face is found in**

**Ans:** Guillain-Barrè syndrome

**184. Atrophy of sternomastoid muscles is found in**

**Ans:** Myotonic dystrophy

**185. Epileptic seizures found in children are called as**

**Ans:** Petit mal

**186. Which phase of epilepsy associated with cyanosis?**

**Ans:** Tonic Phase

**187. Bacteria isolated from cerebral abscess in immuno-compromised patient is**

**Ans:** Streptococcus milleri

**188. Which is the main clinical features of Parkinson's disease?**

**Ans:** Bradykinesia

**189. Mild form of Parkinson's disease can be managed by**

**Ans:** Trihexyphenidyl

**190. Increased incidence of enamel defects in children is found in**

**Ans:** Cerebral palsy

**191. In Bell's palsy, food is retained in upper and lower buccal and labial folds due to weakness of which muscle?**

**Ans:** Buccinator muscle

**192. Which is the initial clinical sign in myasthenia gravis?**

**Ans:** Diplopia and ptosis

**193. Gingival hyperplasia induced by phenytoin first starts in**

**Ans:** Interdental papillae

**194. Which virus is not related to onset of insulin dependent diabetes mellitus?**

**Ans:** Epstein-Barr virus

**195. Rapid weight loss with salt and water depletion is found in**

**Ans:** Type 1 diabetes

**196. The clinical features of type 2 diabetes are?**

**Ans:** Chronic fatigue and malaise

**197. Burning sensation in soles of feet in diabetic patient is caused due to**

**Ans:** Peripheral neuropathy

**198. Which is the pathognomonic oral manifestation of diabetes?**

**Ans:** Median rhomboid glossitis

**199. Dry socket after tooth extraction in diabetic patients in caused due to**

**Ans:** Atherosclerosis

**200. What is the rare oral manifestation of diabetes mellitus?**

**Ans:** Xanthoma

**201. In diabetic patients, what precautions are mandatory for complicated oral procedures in dental emergencies?**

**Ans:** Complicated oral procedures should be avoided and performed on stabilization of blood glucose level

**202. Increase in absolute neutrophil count above 30,000/ mm3 is called as**

**Ans:** Leukemoid reaction

**203. Oral ulcers characterized by necrosis and without surrounding inflammation are found in**

**Ans:** Neutropenia

**204. The large, irregular, foul smelling oral ulcers surrounded by pale mucosa are found in**

**Ans:** Leukemia

**205. Pel-Ebstein fever is found in which disease?**

**Ans:** Hodgkin's disease

**206. Fast-growing, painless, bluish, soft masses on palate which may ulcerate are found in?**

**Ans:** Non-Hodgkin's lymphoma

**207. Multiple myeloma is characterized by**

**Ans:** Amyloidosis of tongue

**208. Purplish red discoloration of oral mucosa is observed in**

**Ans:** Primary polycythemia

**209. What should be minimum concentration of haemoglobin in iron deficiency anemia to administer general anesthesia?**

**Ans:** 10 g/dl and 12 g/dl

**210. Delayed eruption and hypoplasia of dentition is found in**

**Ans:** Sickle cell anemia

**211. The color of skin in patients with thalassemia is ashen-gray due to**

**Ans:** Jaundice, pallor and hemosiderosis

**212. The most frequent oral manifestation in Cooley's (Thalassemia major) anemia is**

**Ans:** Bimaxillary protrusion

**213. "Beefy red" tongue with erythematous areas is found in**

**Ans:** Pernicious anemia

**214. Spontaneous haemorrhage from gingiva is characteristic features of**

**Ans:** Aplastic anemia

**215. Patient complains of "spasm in the throat" in**

**Ans:** Plummer-Vinson syndrome

**216. Which is the characteristic clinical feature of polycythemia vera?**

**Ans:** Cyanosis of face, varicosities in tongue and pruritus

**217. Hypopigmentation of skin and hair is found in which syndrome?**

**Ans:** Chèdiak-Higashi syndrome

**218. The most common oral infection in leukemic patients is of**

**Ans:** Candidiasis

**219. The most common cause of oral ulcerations in leukemic patients on chemotherapy is**

**Ans:** Herpes simplex virus infections

**220. The etiology of Burkitt's lymphoma is most closely linked with**

**Ans:** Epstein-Barr virus

**221. Clinical test used to evaluate primary hemostasis is**

**Ans:** Platelet count

**222. The normal level of circulating fibrinogen is**

**Ans:** 250 mg/dl

**223. Hemophilia A is caused by deficiency of**

**Ans:** Antihemophilic factor

**224. Prolonged bleeding after tooth extraction in patients with haemophilia A is seen when level of factor VIII is**

**Ans:** 7%–50% of normal

**225. Microvascular infracts in gingiva and other mucosal surfaces are found in**

**Ans:** Thrombotic thrombocytopenic purpura

**226. Mild moderate haemophilia A can be managed by administration of**

**Ans:** Desmopressin acetate

**227. Which oral structure exhibits most frequently bleeding in haemophilia?**

**Ans:** Labial frenum

**228. Which oral manifestations occur in hemophilic patient?**

**Ans:** Bleeding from buccal mucosa, severe periodontal disease and TMJ arthropathy

**229. The management of thrombocytopenia includes**

**Ans:** Transfusion of platelets, plasma exchange therapy and corticosteroids

**230. Excessive bleeding caused due to anticoagulant medication such as heparin, during surgical procedure can be managed by administration of**

**Ans:** Protamine sulphate

**231. Chronic abnormal bleeding in uremic patients can be treated by**

**Ans:** Conjugated estrogen preparation and recombinant erythropoietin

**232. Oral hemorrhages related to thrombocytopenia, associated with chemotherapeutic drugs, can be managed by**

**Ans:** Transfusions of HLA matched platelets

**233. Disseminated intravascular coagulation can be treated by administration of**

**Ans:** Intravenous heparin

**234. Which drug inhibits fibrinolysis by blocking the conversion of plasminogen to plasmin?**

**Ans:** Tranexamic acid

**235. Treatment of pharyngeal gonorrhoea includes administration of**

**Ans:** Single dose of ceftriaxone 125–250 mg IM

**236. Reiter's disease is caused by**

**Ans:** Chlamydia trachomatis

**237. Slightly raised grayish white oral lesions surrounded by an erythematous base found in syphilis are known as**

**Ans:** Mucous patches

**238. Oral manifestations of tertiary syphilis are**

**Ans:** Paresthesia in the lips and tongue

**239. "Syphilitic rhagades" near the angle of the mouth are found in**

**Ans:** Congenital syphilis

**240. Oral manifestations of congenital syphilis are characterized by**

**Ans:** "Peg-shaped" incisors and "Mulberry molar"

**241. Donovan bodies are found in cytological examination of**

**Ans:** Granuloma inguinale

**242. The recommended dose of acyclovir for the treatment of oropharyngeal HSV infection is**

**Ans:** 200 mg five times daily

**243. Oral ulcerations with pharyngitis, tonsillitis and cervical lymphadenopathy are found in**

**Ans:** Infectious mononucleosis

**244. Oral condyloma acuminatum can be treated by**

**Ans:** Surgical excision, cryotherapy and $CO_2$ laser therapy

**245. Isolated mucosal ulcers with membranous gingivostomatitis are the clinical features of**

**Ans:** Gonococcal stomatitis

**246. Ulcerative gingivostomatitis with sore mouth are the clinical features of**

**Ans:** Herpetic stomatitis

**247. Extensive superficial ulceration on the lip with a well-defined elevated granulomatous margin is found in**

**Ans:** Granuloma inguinale

**248. Dysphagia and red soft palate with regional lymphadenopathy are the oral manifestations of**

**Ans:** Lymphogranuloma venereum

**249. Pharyngitis, perioral vesicular rash with acute gingivostomatitis are the clinical features of**

**Ans:** Oropharyngeal HSV infection

**250. Age-related changes in the oral-mucosa of an older individual is/are**

**Ans:** Delayed wound healing, dry mucosa and loss of elasticity

**251. Pigmented lesions common in elderly people are**

**Ans:** Melanotic macules

**252. Oral vesiculobullous disease that primarily affects older women is**

**Ans:** Cicatricial pemphigoid

**253. The most common viral infection in older persons is of**

**Ans:** Varicella-zoster virus

**254. Root surface caries in elderly individuals may be caused due to**

**Ans:** Gingival recession, salivary gland hypofunction and orofacial motor deficits

**255. Which oral disease may produce desquamative gingivitis?**

**Ans:** Cicatricial pemphigoid

**256. Which is not an intraoral sequelae of insufficient salivary production in older individuals?**

**Ans:** Candidiasis in the labial commissures

**257. Postherpetic neuralgia in older patients can be treated by administration of**

**Ans:** Analgesics and tricyclic antidepressants

**258. Which drug can be prescribed in salivary gland infection until its culture and sensitivity report is received?**

**Ans:** Amoxicillin

**259. Recommended dose of pilocarpine for the treatment of salivary hypofunction in older patients is**

**Ans:** 5–7.5 mg three times daily

**260. Pilocarpine and cevemeline are contraindicated for patients with**

**Ans:** Pulmonary diseases

**261. Which systemic conditions are associated with microbial infections in elderly patients?**

**Ans:** Immunosuppression, steroid therapy and radiation sequelae

**262. Which drugs commonly prescribed in older patients may lead to lichenoid mucosal lesions?**

**Ans:** Thiazide diuretics

**263. Name various types of radiations**

**Ans:** Wave-like and electromagnetic radiations

**264. Factors necessary for the production of X-rays are**

**Ans:** Source of electrons, accelerator and target

**265. When a photon interacts with an orbiting electron, imparting some of its energy to it, and dislodges it, the process is called**

**Ans:** Compton scattering

**266. The unit of measurement of radiation exposed to the patients during dental X-ray procedure is the**

**Ans:** Roentgen

**267. The unit of measuring X-radiation absorbed from the radiation beam per unit mass of tissue is**

**Ans:** Rad/gray

**268. The SI unit of measuring radioactivity is**

**Ans:** Becquerel

**269. Hypoxic conditions are**

**Ans:** More radioresistant

**270. The most radiosusceptible organ for radiation cancer is**

**Ans:** Stomach

**271. The base of dental X-ray film is composed of**

**Ans:** Polyester polyethylene terephthalate

**272. 'EMULSION' in the X-ray film consists of**

**Ans:** Gelatin and silver halide

**273. What are the numbers of periapical and bitewing films required in full mouth radiographic examination?**

**Ans:** 14 Periapical and 4 bitewing

**274. Higher the value of 'grid ratio'**

**Ans:** Higher is the film contrast

**275. The 'grid-ratio' preferred for optimum image contrast is**

**Ans:** 8–10

**276. Intensifying screen is composed of**

**Ans:** Base, titanium oxide, phosphor and protective coat

**277. How many centres of rotation are there in orthopantomograph?**

**Ans:** Three centres of rotation

**278. Removal of less penetrating X-rays during radiography is known as**

**Ans:** Filtration

**279. The islands of necrotic bone within the radiolucent area is indicative of**

**Ans:** Osteomyelitis

**280. 'The branchless fruit laden tree' is characteristic appearance of**

**Ans:** Sjögrens syndrome

**281. 'Cotton wool' appearance is characteristic radiographic feature of**

**Ans:** Osteomyelitis and Paget's disease

**282. In 'eosinophilic granuloma', affected tooth/teeth appear radiographically as**

**Ans:** Standing in space (Floating teeth)

**283. The most common site for the occurence of Nasopalatine canal cyst is**

**Ans:** Maxillary central incisors

**284. 'Nasopalatine cyst' appears radiographically as**

**Ans:** Heart-shaped

**285. 'Naso-alveolar cyst' appears radiographically as**

**Ans:** Not apparent on radiograph

**286. 'Soap-bubble' appearance is the characteristic feature of**

**Ans:** Ameloblastoma

**287. 'Adenomatoid odontogenic tumor' is commonly associated with**

**Ans:** Unerupted tooth

**288. Name a chemical added in developer for developing a dental radiograph**

**Ans:** Sodium thiosulphate

**289. Radiolucencies of the jaw may not be seen in**

**Ans:** Hypoparathyroidism

**290. X-rays were discovered by**

**Ans:** Roentgen

**291. What type of charges does X-ray have?**

**Ans:** Neutral

**292. Velocity of X-ray is**

**Ans:** Equal to that of light

**293. Which tissue is not imaged by MRI?**

**Ans:** Bone

**294. Number of intensifying screens in film holding cassette is/are**

**Ans:** Two

**295. 'Osteoma cutis' is the soft tissue ossification, of**

**Ans:** Skin

**296. 'Transpharyngeal projection' is required for viewing**

**Ans:** Lateral surface of condylar head and neck

**297. 'Reverse Towne's projection' is required for viewing**

**Ans:** Posterior aspect of both condylar heads and necks

**298. Function of Potter-Bucky diaphragm is**

**Ans:** To absorb scattered radiations

**299. What is used in xeroradiography?**

**Ans:** Selenium Plate

**300. Reason for insufficient image contrast may be**

**Ans:** Excessive peak kilovoltage

**301. Reason for dark radiographs may be**

**Ans:** High temperature of developer, high concentration of developer and inadequate fixation

**302. CT number represents**

**Ans:** A calculation of actual attenuation of the X-ray beam by the body

**303. Hypercementosis is associated which bone disease?**

**Ans:** Paget's disease

**304. What type of radiographic appearance is associated with the osteosarcoma?**

**Ans:** Sun-ray spicules appearance

**305. The dentigerous cyst is always associated with the**

**Ans:** Crown of unerupted tooth

**306. How 'incisive foramen' and 'granuloma' can be differentiated radiographically?**

**Ans:** Lamina dura shows discontinuity in granuloma

**307. Name few structures which appear radiopaque in radiographs?**

**Ans:** Nasal septum, genial tubercle and tooth-crypts

**308. On radiograph mental foramen may be confused as**

**Ans:** Radicular cyst

**309. The height of safe light from the working area should be**

**Ans:** 1.22 meter (4 feet)

**310. Temperature of X-ray processing tanks should be**

**Ans:** Between 60° F–75° F

**311. Name the metal that is radiopaque?**

**Ans:** Lead

**312. What will happen if film will be exposed to natural light or very close to red light during development?**

**Ans:** The film will be dark

**313. Which lesion involves single bone?**

**Ans:** Central giant cell granuloma

**314. For a patient suspected with multiple myeloma, which radiographic views are required to confirm the diagnosis?**

**Ans:** Lateral skull view and anteriorposterior view

**315. Name the odontogenic tumor that does not show radiopacity**

**Ans:** Ameloblastic fibroma

**316. Maxillary sinus is best viewed in which type of radiograph?**

**Ans:** Water's view (or occipitomental view)

**317. 'Cervical burnout' is seen in periapical and bitewing view of**

**Ans:** Intact promixal root surface of premolars

**318. 'Disinfectant' used for infection control during radiography is/are**

**Ans:** Iodophors, chlorines and phenols

**319. Delayed eruption of teeth is seen in**

**Ans:** Cleidocranial dysostosis

**320. 'Radiology' may be defined as**

**Ans:** Science and art of production of X-rays, and their applications to medicine and dentistry

**321. X-rays were discovered in**

**Ans:** 1895

**322. 'Cathode' in a X-ray tube is made up of**

**Ans:** Tungsten

**323. What is the function of 'Cathode' in a X-ray tube?**

**Ans:** To expel the electrons from the circuit and focus them in the focal spot of anode in form of beam

**324. 'Anode' in a X-ray tube is made up of**

**Ans:** Tungsten embedded in copper stem

**325. Soft X-rays**

**Ans:** Possess less energy, have larger wavelength and have little penetrating power

**326. In the 'developer' sodium sulphite acts as a**

**Ans:** Preservative

**327. The fetus is most susceptible to the radiation-hazards in which stage?**

**Ans:** Stage of organogenesis

**328. Target is kept at an angle of**

**Ans:** 20°

**329. Target is made up of tungsten, because of its**

**Ans:** High melting point, high atomic number and low vapour pressure

**330. Generally, the voltage in a dental X-ray machine is maintained at**

**Ans:** 50–75 kVp

**331. Mostly the shape of collimator is**

**Ans:** Rectangular

**332. 'Oil' is circulated around the X-ray tube to**

**Ans:** Dissipate the heat

**333. 'Hard radiations' are produced by**

**Ans:** Metals of high atomic weight

**334. Radiations produced from focal spots are**

**Ans:** Primary Radiations

**335. Which radiations are reflected from object, are reduced by increasing the grid ratio and reduce the contrast of the image?**

**Ans:** Secondary radiations

**336. X-rays can be concentrated to a desired area by**

**Ans:** Adjusting size and shape of a cone

**337. The tissue most susceptible to radiation is**

**Ans:** Blood forming cells

**338. The function of lead foil in a film packet is**

**Ans:** To absorb secondary radiations

**339. Films should be washed after fixing for at least**

**Ans:** 10 minutes

**340. The function of hydroquinone in a developer solution is**

**Ans:** To increase the contrast of the image

**341. What is the colour of new developer and fixer?**

**Ans:** Clear

**342. What is 'Fluorescence'?**

**Ans:** Emission of visible light by a crystal when subjected to an activating form of energy

**343. Which technique is based on geometrical theorem?**

**Ans:** Bisecting technique

**344. Which disease will not produce radiolucent appearance on radiograph?**

**Ans:** Hypoparathyroidism

**345. 'Pepper-pot skull' is the radiographic feature of**

**Ans:** Hyperparathyroidism

**346. 'Ground glass' appearance is characteristic feature of**

**Ans:** Fibrous dysplasia, hyperparathyroidism and paget's disease

**347. 'Honeycomb appearance' is seen in**

**Ans:** Mucoepidermoid carcinoma, ameloblastoma and central haemangioma

**348. 'Codman's triangle' is the radiographic feature of which bone lesion?**

**Ans:** Osteosarcoma

**349. Which sarcoma shows 'onion-skin effect' on radiograph?**

**Ans:** Ewing's sarcoma

**350. 'Punched-out' radiographic outline describes for**

**Ans:** Outline showing no peripheral bone reaction

**351. On intraoral periapical radiographs which anatomic structures is not recognized?**

**Ans:** Infraorbital foramen

**352. Following acute pulpitis is the first radiographic evidence of apical pathology**

**Ans:** Thickening of the periodontal space

**352. In which year bitewing X-ray film technique was introduced?**

**Ans:** 1925

**353. Radiation protection laws or codes require that the diameter of dental X-ray beams measured at the patient's face should not be of more than**

**Ans:** 6.985 cm (2.75 inch)

**354. X-rays were discovered in**

**Ans:** Germany

**355. In X-ray tube anode is kept at an angle of**

**Ans:** 20°

**356. Anode is made of tungsten because**

**Ans:** High fusing temperature, high atomic number and high thermal conductivity

**357. Bitewing X-rays are especially useful**

**Ans:** To detect initial caries and periodontal lesions.

**358. Which tissue is most susceptible to radiation?**

**Ans:** Basal cells of oral mucosa

**359. Units of X-rays are**

**Ans:** Roentgen

**360. X-ray tubes are immersed in oil so as to**

**Ans:** Cool the target

**361. Base of an X-ray film is made up of**

**Ans:** Cellulose acetate

**362. Mainly damage to X-ray tube is caused by**

**Ans:** Milliampere

**363. What is colour of exhausted (fully used) developer?**

**Ans:** Brown

**364. An occlusal radiograph of maxillary arch shows a relatively large radiolucent area between the roots of the right lateral incisor and the right canine. The roots of both teeth are displaced laterally. Both teeth are vital, the probable diagnosis is**

**Ans:** Globulomaxillary cyst

**365. In a periapical radiograph which anatomic structure most commonly 'is superimposed over the apices of the mandibular premolars and is interpreted as a pathologic condition?**

**Ans:** Mental foramen

**366. The wavelength of X-ray photons is determined by the**

**Ans:** Kilovoltage

**367. In an X-ray machine the purpose of a step-up transformer is to increase the**

**Ans:** Voltage to the tube's anode-cathode circuit

**368. In sickle cell anemia certain radiographic changes in the bone of the skull appear. These changes may be**

**Ans:** "Hair on end" effect

**369. In an 8-year-old child bilateral, asymptomatic, cyst-like radiolucent lesions occurring in the bone at the angles of the mandible are most likely related to a condition called**

**Ans:** Cherubism

**370. Which rays are most likely to be absorbed by the skin and produce an X-ray injury?**

**Ans:** X-rays of long wavelength

**371. Upon living tissues is the basic effect of X-radiation**

**Ans:** Ionization

**372. A globulomaxillary cyst in a periapical radiograph most likely appear that the cyst**

**Ans:** Is located lateral to tooth roots

**373. Intensifying screens in extraoral radiology are used in radiographic examination in order to**

**Ans:** Decrease the exposure

**374. An aluminium disk in the primary X-ray beam is add to**

**Ans:** Reduce long wavelength radiation

**375. The least susceptible tissue of the body to X-radiation, is**

**Ans:** Mature bone

**376. Guide for the radiation protection recommends that the per week X-ray dose to operators of dental X-ray machines should not exceed**

**Ans:** 100 milliroentgens

**377. A periapical radiograph reveals a radiolucent shadow at the apex of the maxillary left central incisor. Lamina dura is continuous and the tooth responds normally to the pulp tester. All clinical signs or symptoms are absent. What is the most probable diagnosis of the radiolucent shadow?**

**Ans:** Normal anatomic landmark

**378. A periapical radiograph of a mandibular lateral incisor reveals a sharp right angle bent of the apical one-third of the root. This is diagnostic of**

**Ans:** Dilacerations

**379. Small roots and obliterated pulp chamber in radiographs of a young adult in permanent teeth are indicative of**

**Ans:** Dentiogenesis imperfect

**380. Presence of multiple to discrete apical radiolucencies in vital, asymptomatic mandibular anterior teeth are mostly suggestive of**

**Ans:** Immature cementomas